the ORDER
of the UNIVERSE

"A mind which is deep and boundless has neither doubts nor thoughts. . . .
To see that the mind is the Tao is to follow the stream and reach the source. . . .
When the meaning has been revealed and the source realized,
words and contemplation do not necessarily remain."

Ch'an Master Yung-Chia (665–713 A.D.)

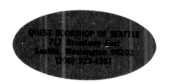

the ORDER
of the UNIVERSE

George Ohsawa

English Version, Introduction, and Notes by Jim Poggi

and
"The Spiralic Concept of Man"
by Herman Aihara

George Ohsawa Macrobiotic Foundation
Oroville, California

Front Cover Photograph: "Miniature Sunflower with Honey Bee"
by Maryanne Caruthers-Akin.

Back Cover: Calligraphy by Korean Zen Master Man'Gong Sunim (1871–1946).
Used with permission of the Zen Lotus Society, Ann Arbor, Michigan.
Silkscreen prints (11″ × 32″) available from the Society, 1214 Packard Road,
Ann Arbor, Michigan 48104.

Map designs by Sue Reid.
Illustrations and calligraphy by Sheri Peterson.

Originally published in Japanese in 1940
First English Edition   1986

Library of Congress Catalog Card Number: 86-82724
ISBN 0-918860-46-6

Preface

To my knowledge, this is the first complete version in English of George Ohsawa's *The Order of the Universe.* I prefer to call it a version rather than a translation. This for two reasons: First, because of its multi-lingual origin. Since I do not read Japanese or French, but know Spanish quite well, I worked from Mauricio Waroquiers' Uruguayan version. I presume that this, in turn, was taken from some French translation or other, which, in its turn, derived from the original Japanese. I am indebted to Herman Aihara for comparing my effort with the Japanese and for making some additions and a number of suggestions both as to content and accuracy of expression. The second reason for calling this a version is that I took certain liberties in expressing what I felt to be the sense of Ohsawa's thought, as opposed to a mere literal rendition. This decision was made in favor of greater clarity and readability.

I am also indebted to Herman Aihara for his support in bringing this version to light, as well as for his willingness to field a number of my questions presented to him along the way. Thanks to fellow staff members Carl Ferre, Sylvia Zuck, and Stan Hodson for suggestions, criticisms, and drudgery gracefully endured. And, finally, I am grateful to my wife, Pat, for her patience and tolerance of my rather long love affair with this book.

Jim Poggi
August 15, 1986

Contents

Introduction

We think back to the pioneers of an earlier century, the
sturdy souls who took their families and their belongings
and who set out into the frontier of the American West.
. . . Today the frontier is space and the boundaries of
human knowledge. . . . We promise Dick Scobee and his
crew that their dream lives on, that the future they
worked so hard to build will become reality. . . . Dick,
Mike, Judy, El, Ron, Greg and Christa, your families and
your country mourn your passing. . . . We can find conso-
lation only in faith, for we know in our hearts that you
who flew so high and so proud now make your home
beyond the stars, safe in God's promise of eternal life.

> – President Ronald Reagan's Memorial Address in
> honor of the crew members of the shuttle *Chal-*
> *lenger,* Houston, January 31, 1986.

Caveat lector! (Reader beware!) What follows is *not* the teaching of
George Ohsawa. It is one interpretation – mine, in this case, written as
an interview – of how Ohsawa might have responded to a contemporary event of international significance, and of how this interpretation
might relate to the content and spirit of this book, Ohsawa's personal
favorite, *The Order of the Universe.* Each reader will undoubtedly bring
his or her own understanding to bear on my own. This is as it should
be, in the spirit of George Ohsawa and the Team of Life Explorers. For
those readers who are not familiar with Ohsawa and his writings I offer
another warning: *Cave canum!* (Watch out! *This* dog bites!) Still, if one
can accept it, an encounter with Ohsawa could transform one's life.

Jim Poggi: First of all, I would like to have your comments on the *Chal-*
lenger disaster.

1

George Ohsawa: [*Imagine a deep, rich, bass, Japanese voice speaking English with a pronounced French accent.*] I would not call it a disaster. Sooner or later, it was bound to happen. It is a sad event for the families of the seven astronauts who died, but really it is a good thing for the United States and for all the other countries of the world.

JP: Will you please explain?

GO: It forces everyone to think and to ask themselves some very important questions. If Mr. Reagan, the Congress, NASA, the techicians, and the astronauts themselves had asked themselves these questions before sending the *Challenger* into space, then perhaps what happened could have been avoided.

JP: I don't understand. What questions?

GO: Ah, it is very obvious to me. The first question must be: "When the spacecraft leaves the launchpad, where does it go?" In other words, "What is its destination? What is this 'dream' the President speaks of in his message?" We all have our dream. In this book I tell you what *my* dream is. Mr. Reagan does not tell us what *his* dream is. In my opinion, he doesn't because he himself doesn't know. He is just speaking words.

JP: But this doesn't make sense. Everyone knows what the dream is: To conquer space, to unravel the mysteries of the solar system and the universe, to tap into new resources that space opens up for us, especially now that the Earth's resources are so depleted.

GO: Such research is ridiculous. We are going into space because we have already destroyed our Planet. Our solar system has already become a junk yard. And next we will be destroying the entire universe.

JP: But what about the so-called "commercialization" of space? Isn't this a good thing? As our population grows, as food and jobs become scarce, don't we need new frontiers to provide fresh opportunities for the world's population?

GO: I respond by reading to you this transcript taken from a news broadcast aired shortly after the shuttle disaster:

> When America's space shuttle roars off the launchpad at Cape Canaveral, it carries the hopes of a nation, who see space as America's last frontier. And it carries the hopes of the business community in this country, who see the commercialization of space as the best business opportunity of the next quarter century. Industry analysts say commercial space can become a trillion-dollar industry by the year 2010. . . . Former astronaut Deke Slayton developed the Conestoga (rocket) and has the first three licenses issued for a private launch. His first customer: a group of funeral homes who promise to launch cremated remains into perpetual orbit. But Slayton says even that launch is two years away, though he does see a bright future for the commercialization of space.
>
> – Newscaster Elizabeth Brackett, The MacNeil/Lehrer News Hour, Houston, February 7, 1986.

I would like to ask Mr. Reagan some questions: "Why are you spending so many dollars and risking lives in your space program? For what did the seven brave young men and women give their lives?" Maybe it was so that rich people could satisfy their desire to be remembered by paying to have their remains sent into space. What do you think? You see, Mr. Reagan and the American people who are paying for this program believe that there is something out there that they must find. This is their dream. But in fact they will find nothing. Such a dream that cannot be realized is pure sentimentality.

JP: That seems like a very harsh judgment.

GO: It may be so, but in this case it is the highest level of judgment. If you don't understand what I say, then you must read this book.

JP: I have, and what struck me right off was your description in Chapter I of the Team of Life Explorers making their way up the River of

Life. If you were writing this book today, I am wondering if you would have changed your team to one of "Space Explorers."

GO: Yes, in the sense that I would have used space instead of a river as my background. I would have painted the picture of space exploration to make my point, since today even young children can understand it. Many people today do not have the opportunity to explore a beautiful river. . . . But it is all the same. You see, it is only natural for everyone to explore. Life itself is the biggest adventure. We are – how do you say? – "as curious as a cat." If man were not curious, he could not survive; he could not anticipate natural disasters or the attacks of an enemy. So it is good that Mr. Reagan and his team of experts are so eager to explore.

JP: But you just said that our space program was a mistake. Now you are saying that it is a good thing to explore the beyond.

GO: If you will recall from reading my book, I told you what the problem is. It is only natural to explore, but to explore you must have eyes. You must see where you are going. Mr. Reagan and his team do not have good eyes. They are very nearsighted. If you are nearsighted and drive a car, you will crash. If you don't want to crash, you must have good eyesight.

JP: A little earlier you said, in referring to space, that there was nothing out there to be found.

GO: That is correct. There is nothing out there that is not on this Earth. Perhaps scientists will discover new elements that do not exist on this Earth, but they will just be more elements and the physicists will just fit them into their charts. They will not find anything else.

JP: Back in the sixties an Anglican priest by the name of John Robinson wrote a disturbing book called *Honest to God*. If I recall correctly, the main thrust of the book was that, if we were looking for God "out there," we were "barking up the wrong tree," if you'll excuse me for mixing a metaphor.

GO: [*Laughing.*] Yes, very good! I agree with the Reverend Robinson. Perhaps Mr. Reagan and his team are looking for God, yes? What did he say in his speech?: " . . . We know in our hearts that you who flew so high and so proud now make your home beyond the stars." These are beautiful words, but I don't think that the astronauts will find God out there. . . . So, I have another question for you brought up by Mr. Reagan himself: "Where did the seven astronauts go after their ship blew up under them? Where is this home beyond the stars that Mr. Reagan speaks of?" I would like to know the answers to these things. Perhaps you can tell me.

JP: The day after the funeral of my first wife, Emily, I thought I saw her in the clouds as I stood on the top of Fremont Peak. Several years later on her anniversary I had the same experience as I looked out at a Mexican sunset. I know that she really wasn't there in the clouds physically, but still, somehow I experienced her presence as the light of the clouds entered my body.

GO: That is just what I am saying. You were not looking for her and she came to you. This is because of your dream, your wish to remain close to her. In this case your eyesight was clear and you saw her. But if you had tried to force her to come to you, she would not have come. To do such a thing is being nearsighted. Mr. Reagan and his team speak of "conquering" space. This is a very narrow (yang) position and is natural to a nation of meat-eaters. It is the same extreme yang energy that has already destroyed our Earth. You need only to look at the results of all the great explorations of the past five centuries, since the time of Christopher Columbus. There is no place in the world that has not suffered from these explorations. As Hitler said: "Today Europe, tomorrow the World!" It is the same thing.

JP: I see your point, but isn't this a very pessimistic view of the state of things?

GO: Oh, no! I am never pessimistic. On the contrary, always I am the eternal optimist. I believe we are living on the edge of a great discovery, one that I have already explained at length in this book. It is a discovery that will save the world, even if atomic war comes. It is my teaching of the Unique Principle, which is only now beginning to be understood.

JP: I think I understand the general idea of this principle, but it would be helpful to me, and perhaps to others, if you would summarize it for me in just a few words.

GO: If you look at the maps which the Team of Life Explorers made, which you will find on pages 29–31, you can understand. It is not a new teaching. It is what all the great teachers of mankind have always taught, as I point out in my book. Today, however, almost everyone is either blind or nearsighted, so they cannot see this teaching clearly. The problem is that they think they see when they don't. And so they continue to look for their god in space.

JP: But you still haven't explained it.

GO: If I did, you would either say that you understood it or that you didn't. If you said you understood it, I would not believe you because you would only be saying that you understood my words. If you said that you did *not* understand it, I would believe you and I would congratulate you. Did not your Great Teacher say, "You are not far from the Kingdom of Heaven?"

JP: This is all very frustrating. I am used to having explanations. When I studied philosophy and theology, I relied on my mental powers to grasp the principles that were being taught. And I, too, used the same method when I gave my sermons or classes. The way you are talking, I really don't understand anything.

GO: That is why I say you are not far from the Kingdom. I name my schools "Les Centres Ignoramus" because only those who know they do not know are capable of understanding this teaching. You Westerners want to understand the words, but you don't realize that they are just words. You mistake the words for the reality. You build a space ship and everyone congratulates you on how perfect and beautiful it is. "Oh, such a wonderful machine!" Then you say that the *Challenger* is ready to go. Only it blows up and seven lives are wasted. Mr. Reagan and his team do not know the Unique Principle. If they did, then they would understand that they do not know everything and would discover their mistakes. But first they must know where they are going. If you will look at the map, you will see that they could only go as far as the Fourth World, the world of Sky. But this is a very nearsighted view of the world. If you cannot see where you are going, you invite disaster.

JP: You will recall that Christa McAuliffe, the thirty-seven-year-old teacher and mother of two, was riding the shuttle when it exploded. After she joined the space program, she was quoted as saying: "What are we doing here? We're reaching for the stars." Do you have any comment on this?

GO: This is a very good example of what I am saying. What is this talk of reaching for the stars? In my opinion it is pure sentimentality. It has nothing to do with true discovery. Why? Because Mrs. McAuliffe does not see beyond the stars to the infinite, eternal, and unchanging world. It is a very limited view of reality.

JP: I was interested to learn that Mrs. McAuliffe had attended a Catholic high school and had been a practicing Catholic. Perhaps her priest . . .

GO: Priests and ministers do not know where they are going either. They speak of God, looking for him in their words and books, not understanding that all that is only of the relative, limited world. Did not Jesus accuse the priests of his day of serving the gods of money and power? Perhaps it is no different today. As I say in this book: "Even were we to consult those teachers – ministers, priests, and preachers – whose business it is to study matters of the Spirit, we still could not depend on their reply, given over, as most of them are, to the over- whelming influence of people and scientists only interested in length, weight, and duration." So priests and ministers, too, must study the Unique Principle so they can teach it to their people. They must read this book.

JP: There are some people who would accuse you of being arrogant. You have strong opinions about things and sometimes your ideas seem outlandish and preposterous. How can you possibly expect to maintain credibility with people when you criticize them so strongly?

GO: Ah, a very good question! Such accusations only make life more interesting and amusing. They are – how do you say? – the "spice of life." Still, those who make such criticisms do so because they cannot accept the teachings of the Unique Principle. They, too, are nearsighted and only see what exists in this relative, changing world. I am happy when such people criticize me because their criticisms tell me that they are questioning their own limited views. Then perhaps some day they may wake up with a clear vision, with eyes that can see into Infinity, into that unchanging, eternal world which you Westerners call God.

JP: You seem to be saying that your students must experience for themselves what you teach. If it's not from your words, which many either reject or fail to understand, then how will they comprehend it?

GO: My work is to ask many questions, to make people think. You are mistaken if you think I am giving you some thoughts and that these thoughts will change you. No one can do that, not even Jesus, or Buddha, or Mohammed. Look how many people have been murdered and how many wars have been waged over the centuries in the name of these teachers. Many sick people walk away from my teachings, even though they could be healed if they accepted them. However, there are no guarantees. All I can tell you is: "Not this! Not that! Not the other thing, either!" It is like I am taking a toy away from you. You want to hold on to your toy because you do not want to grow up and take responsibility. So I grab your toy and take it away from you. This is what I do with my words. And so you cry and scream like a spoiled child. But maybe you will let go of the toy and see the Truth.

JP: But isn't it a matter of your ideas versus other people's ideas and opinions? By doing this don't you set yourself up so that people reject your teachings?

GO: You don't understand. What I teach are not opinions. I teach only the Unique Principle of yin and yang in the relative world. There is absolutely no change in my teaching that in this relative world everything changes. There is no one who can refute this teaching. I say that everything we know is of this relative world, including the so-called findings of modern science. I say that the materialistic thinking of science is nearsighted because it sets itself up as a god and invites people to worship at its feet. But in order to justify its pretensions science must deposit God out there in space somewhere, claiming that we must set out to find him. This is the pie in the sky.

JP: Your position seems to me to be one of agnosticism. Are you saying that we cannot know anything but a relative, changing, and unstable world? That we cannot know God?

GO: Ah, ha! You are getting warmer. You must not look for God out there, nor within the human heart, either. The furthest star is still in space, which is of the relative, changing world. Your heart, too, occupies space. How can God be found in space if space is of the relative world?

JP: But then where is God to be found?

GO: Maybe you will find Him by reading my book? [*Laughs.*] Anyway, you are on the right track. But I want to go back to your heart. Although it occupies space, was it not your great St. Augustine who said, "Our hearts were made for you, Oh God, and they are ever restless until they find their rest in you?"

JP: So?

GO: Your heart beats so many times per minute, sometimes more, sometimes less. That is why Augustine calls the heart restless, because it never rests. If it rests, you will die. [*Laughing.*] Maybe thanks to St. Augustine we have unwittingly discovered a new proof for the existence of God, equal to the five proofs of St. Thomas Aquinas. Only ours is much easier to understand: If your heart is restless, then, according to the principle of yin and yang, there must be Someone or Somewhere where the heart can rest, and that is God!

JP: I am surprised in talking with you and in reading your book to hear you speaking so often about God. I don't recall having seen the word "God" in your other writings. Would you explain?

GO: Oh yes, that is very simple. Sometimes people ask me if I believe in God. I always answer "no." "No, I do not *believe* in God." The great teachers of the Orient and of the West, for that matter, have never believed in God. I do not believe in God, because I know him. For me, God is the same as the Unique Principle, the absolute, infinite, and eternal world. If you truly understand this, and if you follow the principles of macrobiotics, then you will be always happy and healthy and free from all fear. This is the great adventure of life.

Journey up the River of Life

The River of Life – what we call "our world" or "our life" – is not just any river one might find in a geography book. This river is so big we have trouble making out its banks. The rocks we see protruding from its surface like tiny islands are called people's "lives." In this river one finds all conceivable kinds of living things. So huge is it that viewed from one of these tiny rock-islands it seems hardly to be moving at all, while in fact it is surging along at a tremendous speed. Everything in this river is moving along night and day. Almost no one has ever attempted to pit himself against this mighty current and move up the River of Life. All scientists have done is to study some insignificant details about some rock or plant found on one of its islands. It seems to me that it is too difficult an undertaking for them to study the river itself.

I invite you to join me in traveling up this River of Life and with me to reach its source.

As our point of departure we need to ask: Where does our physical life come from? We know, of course, that it is passed on to us by our parents and forebears. But, what is the origin of our parents' lives and how have those lives been maintained? The answer is not so difficult since we know there are many factors involved. But the most important of these is food. Food is the very basis of our lives. It is thanks to food that we are alive at all. Without food we wouldn't be able to live, think, or propagate. The only way to discover the profound meaning of food in our lives and its great and mysterious power is to fast. I recommend fasting to those who haven't yet undertaken it as an experiment.

Over the course of thousands of years it is thanks to food that man has been born, has produced offspring, has lived, been active, thought, created, mastered ideas, and known God. Thinking about it this way we can understand how food is the origin of life. Our bodies are a trans- formation of the food we eat. There is vegetal and animal food, water too, and the nourishment provided by the air and the sun's light.

Of these sources of food, vegetal foods are the main ones since all animals, including man, live by eating grains and vegetables either directly or indirectly. Grains and vegetables have no capacity to move themselves, but they give rise to those creatures, namely man and animals, who do enjoy this ability of self-locomotion. So what moves comes from that which does not move. It could be that Newton got this far up the River of Life, when he demonstrated that all bodies impelled by an initial force will move infinitely in the direction of that force provided that no contrary motion or obstacle intervenes.[1] In my opinion, that initial force (as well as the obstacle) is the source of the River of Life. In short, the origin of animal life is the vegetal world, our first support base.

What, then, is the origin of the vegetal world? It is the Earth, our second support base. The Earth is made up of soil and water. And the soil contains all the various minerals. The Earth spins incessantly, not stopping even for a second. What does not move (the vegetal world) arises from what does move (the Earth). Still, the mere existence of the vegetal world and of soil and water is not enough to account for the existence of animal life; similarly, the vegetal world does not exist by the Earth alone.

The Earth, too, cannot exist of and by itself. Necessary to its existence as well as to that of the vegetal and animal worlds is the Sky,[2] whose covering of air enshrouds the Earth like a mantel. The Sky does not move. A moving Earth is born of an immovable Sky. And so the Sky becomes our third support base.

Still, man and animals cannot live only by the supports we have so far mentioned. We need something more: the Light of the sun, which is heat, the source of fire. Without Light neither the Sky, nor the Earth, nor the vegetal or animal and human worlds would be capable of existence. Truly, from this Light is born the Sky, a light that moves at a tremendous velocity. The Sky, which does not move, is born of that which moves, the Sun, our fourth support base. So far we have discovered four elements which support the animal and vegetal worlds, namely, Earth, Water, Wind (Sky), and Fire.[3] These four elements the great Greek and Indian philosophers already knew.

Have we now arrived at the wellspring of life? No, something is still missing. Even supposing our bodies could live by these four elements, still, lacking Spirit, they would be nothing but living corpses. But what is the origin of Spirit? By what is it nourished and how does it develop? A body in which the Spirit does not dwell cannot be a living body. A body has length (centimeters), weight (grams), and duration (seconds). It is visible, maintains a certain temperature, and moves. But Spirit doesn't manifest any of these particular qualities. Could Spirit, then, be the origin of the four elements? This is the question we shall be exploring. In any case, we know Spirit doesn't have length, weight, or time.

Scientists don't consider it worth their while taking a look at anything they can't perceive with their senses. And so it's a waste of time to question them as to the nature of Spirit. Even were we to consult those teachers – ministers, priests, and preachers – whose business it is to study matters of the Spirit, we still could not depend on their reply, given over as most of them are to the overwhelming influence of the materialistic thinking of people and scientists only interested in length, weight, and time. With even greater reason we could say that the answer is not to be found among politicians and educators.

Let us clarify the meaning of Spirit. We cannot know Spirit by way of the five senses. Whereas the body weakens with age, the Spirit never grows old. One has the impression that even in advancing years it has the naiveness or innocence of a child. What increases or decreases in relation to the body is of the physical order and does not touch the Spirit. Since it lacks form, the Spirit does not age; neither does it suffer growth or decline. On the other hand, our bodies, our thinking, our experiences, and so on, are all of the limited, finite order. How great is this Spirit of ours? Where are we to find it?

Some have held that the Spirit is in the heart or in the head or at the body's core. These are very strange ideas. A dead body will still have a heart and a stomach and a head, but the Spirit will not be found in any of these. Maybe it's that the Spirit enters the body and then leaves it again? But no one has ever seen this. Besides, Spirit has no form. The problem it presents to us is that it is invisible. Still, throughout all of history people have believed in its existence even though it would seem not to dwell in the body. To catch this Spirit is truly a task of enormous proportions. If only we could somehow grasp it.

First of all, we think about Spirit as being opposed to matter, believing that matter is within the power of our understanding. However, to tell the truth, it isn't. They say that a substance is made up of some hundreds of elements, each element being composed of electrons and protons. But no one knows what *these* in turn are made of. All the more reason for accepting the fact that we don't understand anything about Spirit. Do we then have no key at all for unlocking its mysteries?

There is one key available to us: *thinking*. Spirit is made manifest through thinking. Thinking is a characteristic of man. We may not know the origin of the electron, but we know that thoughts exist.[4] While asleep we don't know where we are or what we are doing. Neither do we know if the *ego* exists or not. Nevertheless, it would seem that the world of thought and the faculty of thinking exist even when we sleep since we are capable of dreaming, and in my opinion thinking is the same as dreaming. But you may say that dreams are irrational and at times absurd. That's why we often say that an incoherent statement is like a dream. But it's quite evident that incoherent, irrational, and absurd thoughts exist even in thinking. As you know, a certain well-known philosopher has said, "Then life is just a dream, or is it the other way around, that the dream is life?"[5]

I would like to make a distinction between irrational dreams and real dreams. In the case of real dreams we perceive events that are at this very moment happening in some far-off place, or we foresee some event that lies in the future. For example, many people while on a trip have the experience of suddenly stopping and exclaiming: "Why, I've seen this place somewhere before!" One remembers having seen it in a dream.

A presentiment too can be classified as a *real* dream. It is a dream dreamed not with the eyes, but with the heart or the Spirit. To me that is why dreaming is like thinking. Some proverbs put it this way: "A saint doesn't dream," or, "If a saint dreamed, his dream would always be real." As for me, I'm neither a saint nor a sage, and at times I have dreams that are absurd. But once in awhile I have a real dream. Especially since taking up the practice of a thoroughgoing macrobiotic way of life I have noticed that my absurd dreams have decreased and my real dreams have increased. Every time I give a lecture I ask my listeners if they can recall any real dreams. I have discovered that all of them have had such dreams, though rarely. I think too that the predictions made by prophets are similar to real dreams.

Dreaming and thinking are strange phenomena. Since I was a child I have always come up with dreams for the future. My first dream in life was to become a novelist. Later I found that I wasn't capable of writing a novel; but then I could at least become a translator. When my mother died, I conceived a great dream of engaging in the fight against disease.

Later on I was particularly drawn to French literature. By way of a very nice dream I fancied going to France some day. In order to realize that dream I found myself wanting to learn French. At the time I was living in such poverty that I couldn't even afford to pay for lessons. Nevertheless, my dreams came true, every one of them. I learned French at a church and paid nothing. I received a travel grant from the Ministry of Agriculture and Commerce and finally set foot on French soil for the first time. After that I visited France many times both as a sailor and in the import business. Finally, I lived in France for ten years promoting an understanding of Japanese culture and the Unique Principle. My dreams were realized one after the other. That's why I ask myself if life is a dream or if, on the contrary, the dream is life.[6]

The first mystery in regard to the real dream is that it has no limits whatsoever. One can dream anything. I once saw an English film "Love Forever" in which two poor lovers, the man tortured day and night in prison and the woman locked in a duke's castle, remained united in their dreams each day in spite of being separated, keeping their love alive until the moment of their deaths. That film made a great impression on me and I came to realize that in England too there is some understanding of the mystery of the dream.[7]

The second mystery that surrounds dreams is that in the real dream sorrows and physical ills do not exist, since we are in the realm of the Unlimited or Absolute. The same may be said of the realm of Spirit. The kinds of sufferings we speak of belong only to the physical world. That is why I believe that the true dream is a manifestation of the Spirit.

We now understand that the special quality of the dream world is that it knows no restrictions; in other words, it is eternal, of a world that transcends both Time and Space. In the realm of the dream one never grows old and one can travel thousands of miles with total ease. Also, both past and present are within the grasp of the dream. In the world of the dream, one is completely free. Is that not a freedom worthy of God?

Many deeds and stories have demonstrated the identity of dream and Spirit. I have already mentioned the film "Love Forever" and the butterfly dream, but even among primitive peoples such as the Hottentots, Eskimos, and Fiji Islanders one can find numerous examples of myths that demonstrate how real the dream is and how it opens us to a world that is free and eternal. I for one have from time to time enjoyed the incredible experience of a true dream of mystery.

In his book, *The Primitive Mind,* Levy-Bruhl, President of the French Philosophical Association, demonstrates how the customs of certain primitive populations reflect their belief in the identity of dream and the real world.[8]

Now our task is to search out the relationships between the infinite, free, and eternal world on the one hand, and our finite, lowly, and ephemeral world consisting of Light, Sky, Earth, vegetal and animal realms on the other.

The Eternal World

From time immemorial the sages of the Orient, out of their vast perception of the Order of the Universe, have known that our finite, relative world was conceived by the infinite, eternal and absolute world and is continually nourished by it. They also understood this conception to be the explanation of the source of life.

The following works – the *Heart Sutra*, the *Tao Te Ching*, the *I Ching*, the *Upanishads*, the *Bible*, the *Kojiki*, etc. – all describe systematically, as it were, the Order of the Universe and reveal to us the origin of the world.[9] But modern man does not understand what is written in these books.

When missionaries first came from the West to spread Christianity in Japan, a great lord said to them: "Show me your God." Just as it is impossible to show our dreams to our neighbor, neither can we "show" God. These days most people are myopic or color-blind just like that Japanese lord. But not only these days. Already in the Middle Ages many Westerners were nearsighted. They set to fighting against religions in a bloody and terrifying way, insisting that they be "shown" God and asserting that all that is invisible does not exist.

Recently, for example, I visited the city of Nagasaki where the sad story of the love between a Japanese woman who believed in the eternity of love, and a Dutch naval officer who cruelly abandoned her, is still remembered.[10] In Nagasaki too the story of fifty-four martyrs who were crucified for their Christian beliefs has not been forgotten.[11]

All this is but a single page in the history of the struggle between those who believe the world is infinite and those who think it is finite. To put it another way, it is a war between nearsighted materialists and blind believers. During the conflicts between religion and science in the Middle Ages Galileo was condemned as a heretic, Giordano Bruno was executed, Luther and Calvin were persecuted, and so on. All these events are so incredible that it is difficult for us to imagine they could have happened. Even the unspeakable atrocities of a Hitler or a

Mussolini will, fifty years from now, appear to be nothing more than a faintly written page of history, to all appearances as unreal as a dream.

The knowledge of a Galileo or of a despot like the lord who ordered the Nagasaki executions was limited to the visible, finite, relative and material world, while the infinite world remained closed to them. Even supposing they could have seen the infinite world, they would not have comprehended the relationship that exists between the finite world and the ultimate reality. On the other hand, for Luther, Calvin, the Japanese martyrs, or the priests who tried to convert the Japanese lord, only the infinite world existed, so much so that they closed their eyes to the world of everyday realities. As a result, they couldn't convince the materialists of the importance of the eternal world, just as the materialists couldn't convert the spiritually-minded to their view of the world.

Why are these two views so opposed to each other? Why is one age materialistic and another spiritual? Why is one country one way and another just the opposite? The Unique Principle offers a solution to these questions, for it provides an explanation of the nature of the relationship existing between the relative ("Sein") and ideal ("Sollen") worlds.

We live today in an age where science is king. So let's talk first about science.

Aristotle, the "father" of Western science, divided science into two disciplines, that of the finite, material world (physics) and that of the spiritual world (metaphysics, or source of the material world). To understand the former is not a problem, since it deals with concrete matters and chooses the visible world as its area of exploration, so that the majority select it as their field of study. Or, putting it another way, we could say that the number of nearsighted people is on the rise.

After fifteen to sixteen hundred years of this struggle between the two camps we can say that the materialists have made heavy inroads on their spiritually-minded counterparts. By the nineteenth century science finally attained its Golden Age. But then by the beginning of the twentieth, it is already finding itself in a blind alley.

Max Planck, the father of Quantum theory, says that science has as its goal the study of the world of the senses. Although this world includes Earth, plants, animals, human beings, etc., nevertheless, compared to the absolute world, it is incredibly small, like a particle of dust in the open sea or sky. Even if many other similar particles were to be born and die it would make no difference to the vastness of the sea or sky. The absolute with all its majesty *is* the eternal world. Its name is "ultimate reality." It is vast, infinite, free, unrestricted and eternal. Max Planck has reportedly said that science must also investigate and study this world of ultimate reality. If he did indeed say this, then science has already admitted defeat and has acknowledged an unseen, eternal and infinite world.[12]

Furthermore, there can exist only one eternal or infinite world – not two or more – because if there were two, neither could be infinite or absolute. By the same token, it is erroneous to think of Time and Space as two different realities. Each is another name for the infinite world that generates them. The spiritual world too is one with the Infinite. Finally, we must also admit the identity of the material world with the spiritual. This summation must be our view of the world.[13] In Japanese and Chinese the word "sekai" means infinite time ("se") and space ("kai"), while the word for Universe ("uchu") means infinite time ("u") and space ("chu"); in Buddhist terminology infinite time is given as "mu-ryo-ju" (infinite age), while infinite space is called "mu-hen-ko" (infinite light).

Summarizing, we can understand how the dream is identical with Spirit, and Spirit with Time and Space. But the modern world's view of all this is far from perfect since it does not admit the identity of the material with the spiritual world. Kant and Planck have demonstrated that the eternal world is the foundation of matter and the material world. What is important to understand is the relationship between the material and finite world (the world of man) on the one hand, and the spiritual and infinite world (the world of God) on the other, although right now I don't want to prolong a philosophical discussion of it all. It is enough to say and affirm that, in these given circumstances of today's conflicting views, the finite world, as great and vast as it is, is only an infinitesimal part of the infinite world.

Even those who consider themselves to be atheists, when they get into difficulties, end up begging for God's help when they unconsciously murmur, "My God!"

Great thinkers too who have studied the finite world, like Newton and Planck, vaguely perceived the existence of the eternal world, the world of God, even though they couldn't demonstrate it logically.[14] It's almost as if they end up believing in God in spite of themselves. It seems to me that they are so moved by the great force that emanates from the infinite world.[15]

What makes it possible for us to enjoy the experience of Freedom, Eternity, Infinity in our dreams and reveries? How is it that we can come and go between the two worlds, the one in which we can enjoy the freedoms experienced during times of dreaming and reveries and the other where worry, conflict, struggle, and despair are our companions in the daily rounds of living, seeing, and feeling?

Does not this experience, perhaps, help us to understand the existence of the eternal world, despite its apparent unreality? Is it possible *not* to believe that the infinite world of the Beyond has brought forth our finite and relative world?

From a state of extreme poverty one can attain great wealth. In the same way only "Nothing" brings forth "Being," or to put it another way, the infinite gives birth to the finite.[16]

Even though people may be extremely wealthy, when it comes time for them to set sail for the other shore, they won't be able to "take it with them."

Here on Earth we are faced with an excess of population; in the other world this cannot even be considered to be a problem. Since the beginning of this world, trillions and trillions of beings have been born and have died, and all of them have been received into the other world. It has never been heard that even one of them was refused admittance. That's another way of saying that the realm of Death is also infinite, nothing more than another synonym for the world of Eternity, the Dream, the Spirit.

We are accustomed to use expressions like these: "Death is a return to the Beyond," "To cross over to the Other Side," or, "To return from the Beyond." This way of speaking comes from our conviction that we are citizens of the other world, that we live for a brief moment in this one and then return again to the other. If that were not the case, then the thought of death or of going away and leaving behind a loved one would be unbearable to us. But then it seems to me that death is really not so sad; rather, it is living that is difficult. Sometimes one prefers to die rather than to suffer. While asleep we forget all suffering, sadness, sinfulness, every form of evil. As one French saying goes, "La morte est la soeur du sommeil" ("Death is the sister of sleep").

As a matter of fact, we can suffer, think, and cry only because we are alive. After death there will be no suffering or pains or sorrows of any kind. They say that death is a peaceful, eternal sleep. To me the infinite, absolute world is a place as calm as sleep. In this eternal world we will not be tormented by the sad events of the past. Even if in this infinite world we would be capable of enjoying happy memories of the past, our hearts would be choked by the pure joy of those very memories. Thinking of past sorrows would be even more out of place. For the world of memory too belongs to that vast domain where infinite tranquility reigns. That is to say, the world of forgetting is also infinite.

Forgetting is to memory what death is to life. For one who lives in this finite world, remembering is the vision of the infinite. On the other hand, forgetting is the impossibility of perceiving the infinite world; in other words, he who has already entered into the infinite world, the kingdom of God, or of Death, knows forgetting. We might say that forgetting is the younger brother of Death.[17]

We have come into this world of remembering from the realm of forgetting, and making our way through this finite existence, we return once more to the world of forgetting. Even great men like Buddha, Jesus, and Mohammed (shall we include the powerful of this earth like Napoleon and Hitler?) disappear at last into this realm of forgetting, a place full of infinite calm, that world we call Death. How ephemeral we are! Our destiny is inevitable: "Thou know'st 'tis common; all that lives must die, passing through nature to eternity," "Pride comes before disaster, and arrogance before a fall," "These violent delights have violent ends."[18] All that remains of a boy's smiling face is a weathered skull.

Such is the Order of the Universe. No reason, though, for taking our own lives, as some do in their anguish and despair over the inevitability of death. Rather, we should have a good time and make this passing existence as happy as possible. But such happiness is the good fortune only of those who know where they are going, namely, to that land that gave birth to us all. These folks can have a good time in life, like young people on an outing. They can let themselves run, dance, and sing. Sick people, on the other hand, won't enjoy the trip and it's their own fault they can't. The true cause of illness is desire, which comes from greed, which results, in turn, from ignorance about the Order of the Universe. I, who have counseled some fifteen thousand sick people, say it outright: Desire, greed, blindness of heart, arrogance, and pride – all these are characteristics of the sick. And it all comes from the ignorance and stupidity caused by the cloud that separates us from true Wisdom.

By nature we possess a cloudless Wisdom, given that we are born of that infinite, absolute world which is of God. We are all children of God and citizens of an infinite, absolute world. Forgetting this truth is the cloud that causes us to be sick.

This cloud is created by an education that would have us believe that there exists only this finite, material, incomplete, and ephemeral world. And in truth all human knowledge is criminal in nature if it does not have as its object the infinite, eternal, and absolute reality, namely, God.

Still the average man-of-the-street is in no position to cast stones at such an education. The fact is that only he who knows God's world is qualified to critique such an education and its curriculum. And such a person can and should reveal that infinite world to those who are ignorant of it. For this reason we are out of line if we attack or blame our neighbor. On the contrary, we need blame and criticize only ourselves. And if we find it impossible to do even that, then at least we should ask the infinite and absolute God for help. For we possess a Spirit that is Infinity itself, truly nothing less than God. Therefore, if we ask, nothing is impossible to us.[19] As we have been taught, "To will is to empower," and, "God responds to our perfect sincerity."

It is to be expected that some people see only the finite, material, and visible realities, since this limited world does in fact exist. The true citizens of this Earth are those who can only recognize a relative world where such sayings as the following hold fast: "Prosperity is not without many fears and distastes," and, " . . . the hour is ill which severs those it should unite."[20] Those who acknowledge the infinite world in addition to the finite world must live as strangers in the latter. Or better, they are like tourists and visitors. They really have no right to protest against those who are citizens of the finite realm and who manage its affairs. The former have no choice but to obey the latter without complaint.

And when the inhabitants of this world run into difficulties or dangers, or when they fall exhausted and find themselves in blind alleys

– the finite world is a place of deadends and all of us always and inevit-
ably find ourselves up against the wall, whereas in the infinite world
there are neither fatigue nor obstacles of any kind – then these
strangers from the other land must come to their assistance and lead
them to the infinite world. Until that day comes, our apostles of the
Absolute have only to spend their time in self-reflection and in pledg-
ing and exercising their moral power so as not to lose their place as
citizens of the Infinite and delegates of a spiritual realm. To put it
another way, they have only to dig more deeply into the infinite treasure vein of Happiness.

But let us get back to our theme and review the relationship
between the infinite and finite worlds.

Given that the world of Spirit is infinite, flowing, whole, and free of
all concerns, we might call it the world of God, of the Universe, of the
Way, of Nature. That this infinite and spiritual world has brought forth
the finite and material one is beyond proof. To attempt it is an impossibility similar to a child's inability to prove the legitimacy of its own
birth. There is no way for a child to prove before a court of law that
these two are really his parents. We just have to take it on faith that
our legal parents are really ours. Even if they weren't, there's nothing
to be done about it. And supposing the child conceives an unfounded
doubt about the matter, his parents keep on being his parents just the
same. There's no choice but to believe it. It's like a profession of faith.
Too bad for the person who can't stir up such a faith! Pity the one who
lives only for this finite, material world. He is a willing slave. He is the
builder of his own dungeon where he condemns himself to live.

As for me, I believe that the infinite God created this finite world.
And that the story of Genesis is not a myth born over the course of
milof years, but a living reality this very moment, each day, each hour,
each minute, each second.

Suppose we want to make something – say, paint a picture, fashion
an object, cook a meal, build a house. These are all functions of the
Spirit. All these intentions will soon turn into realities. One who has
the intention of building a comfortable house will one day realize his
dream, that is to say, the house will become a creation of the Spirit.
Without that Spirit a house cannot be built. Thanks to Spirit we can
realize whatever dream we choose in this finite world.

Is this Spirit the same as free will? Is not free will behind the reali-
zation of every dream, of every desire in this limited, material world? If
the dream cannot be realized, it is only because one lacks enough
knowledge about this finite, material, visible world. It's like a man try-
ing to build a stone house without any stones. You can't paint a picture
without canvas and oils. It's of crucial importance to know well this
finite world which God has made. And to know God as well, the creator
of this world.

One often hears it said that Napoleon realized his dream. Perhaps
he knew of the infinite world, the realm of the Spirit. Still he died a
miserable death because he knew the infinite world only in part. In any
case I believe that the infinite world, which I call God, has created this
world, humankind, and civilization. It doesn't matter to me if anyone
else chooses to believe this or not. All a skeptic has is this limited,
material, passing world. But all the same, such a skeptic can be a great
help to me since he will teach me many interesting things about his
world.

We have arrived, finally, at the base of the infinite, invisible, eternal
world. Let's raise our tent here and set up camp.

We explored our way up the River of Life and arrived first at the
vegetal world, source of our nourishment. Moving on from there we
discovered the realm of Earth, entered the vast space of the Sky, and
soon reached its outermost limits. Finally, having traversed the domain
of Light, our River of Life vanished and we realized that beyond this
point lies only the invisible and infinite world, a world without light.
We are filled with a sense of wonder, like the youth who loses himself
on the mountain in search of the source of the stream that wanders by
his house, only to find that it suddenly disappears. And so he doesn't
know what to do, even though he realizes that the rain which falls from
the sky is the true source of his stream.

Rain is only matter originating in the finite world. Later that young
man will understand something of its origin, since it is a finite thing.
But life does not exist without Spirit. That's why it isn't easy to grasp
the meaning of life. In any case, we have arrived, with a child's sense of
wonder, at the conclusion that this invisible world is the Infinite, God,
the Universe, Nature, that it is the Matrix of this finite world, since it
is in itself both infinite and eternal. This invisible world is the world of

mystery. It is beyond Time and Space. It is the realm of infinite time and infinite space. It is "Taikyo-ku",[21] God, Truth, the Infinite. And since it is infinite, it is the Spirit, the Dream, Death, Existence.

Maps Used by the Team of
Life Explorers

The Team of Life Explorers has set up its camp at the epicenter of the infinite world. Since this world is infinite, one is always at its "center," no matter where he may physically be. The team has just written its reports and has drawn sketches of the worlds they have explored. There are just three maps, all simple enough even for a child's understanding.[22]

Each map is made up of six levels defined by five concentric circles.[23] The most inward level is red, the next (proceeding outward) is blue, the next, red, and so on. After drawing these three maps, the explorers disappeared. Probably they emigrated to the infinite world, because it is such a pleasant place to live and there one can enjoy complete freedom. We must then, with the help of these three maps, build a conception of the Universe, a vision of the world, and an understanding of life. But what does all this mean?

MAP I ~ MADE BY THE LIFE EXPLORERS ~

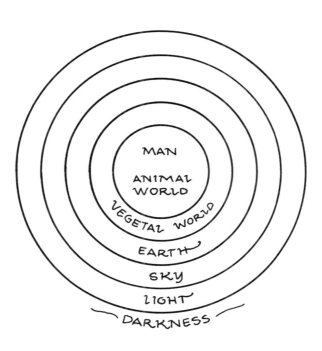

MAP II ~ MADE BY THE LIFE EXPLORERS ~

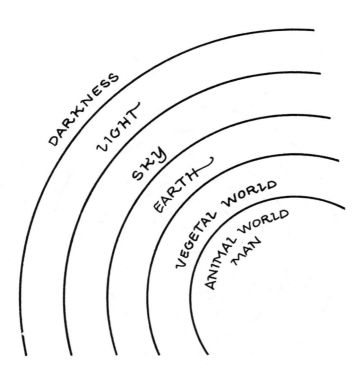

DARKNESS
LIGHT
SKY
EARTH
VEGETAL WORLD
ANIMAL WORLD
MAN

⌐ *Examples of Yin-Yang Order Appearing in the Human World* ⌐

Man and Woman
Body and Spirit
Sadness and Joy
Pleasure and Anger
Love and Hate
Tears and Blood
Happiness and Misfortune
Good and Evil
Left and Right
Controller and the Controlled
6 Yin Organs and 5 Yang Organs
White Blood Cell and Red Blood Cell

Work and Rest
War and Peace
Life and Death
Activity and Sleep
Head and Extremities (Hands/Feet)
Mother and Children
Health and Sickness
Tension and Relaxation
Knowledge and Ignorance
Cold and Hot
Artery and Vein

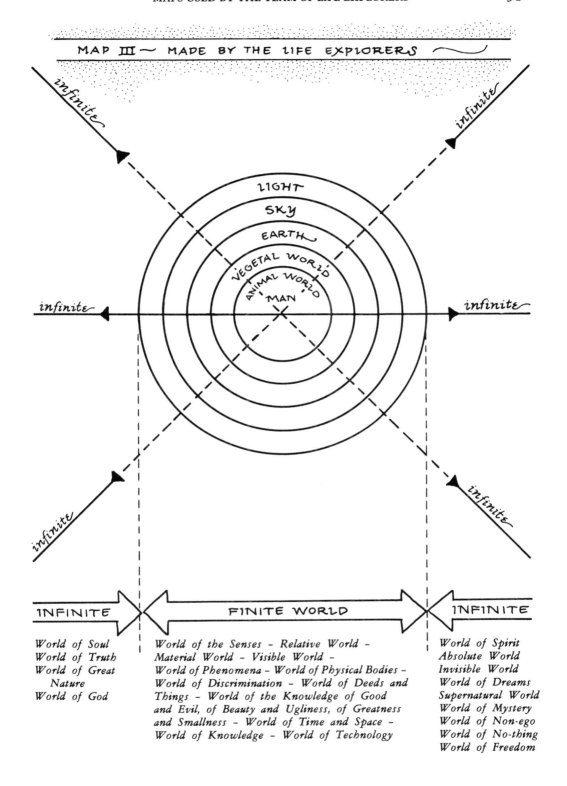

MAP III ~ MADE BY THE LIFE EXPLORERS ~

infinite

infinite

infinite

infinite

infinite

infinite

LIGHT
SKY
EARTH
VEGETAL WORLD
ANIMAL WORLD
MAN

INFINITE — FINITE WORLD — INFINITE

World of Soul
World of Truth
World of Great
    Nature
World of God

World of the Senses - Relative World -
Material World - Visible World -
World of Phenomena - World of Physical Bodies -
World of Discrimination - World of Deeds and
Things - World of the Knowledge of Good
and Evil, of Beauty and Ugliness, of Greatness
and Smallness - World of Time and Space -
World of Knowledge - World of Technology

World of Spirit
Absolute World
Invisible World
World of Dreams
Supernatural World
World of Mystery
World of Non-ego
World of No-thing
World of Freedom

MAP IV ~ CONSTITUTION OF THE UNIVERSE

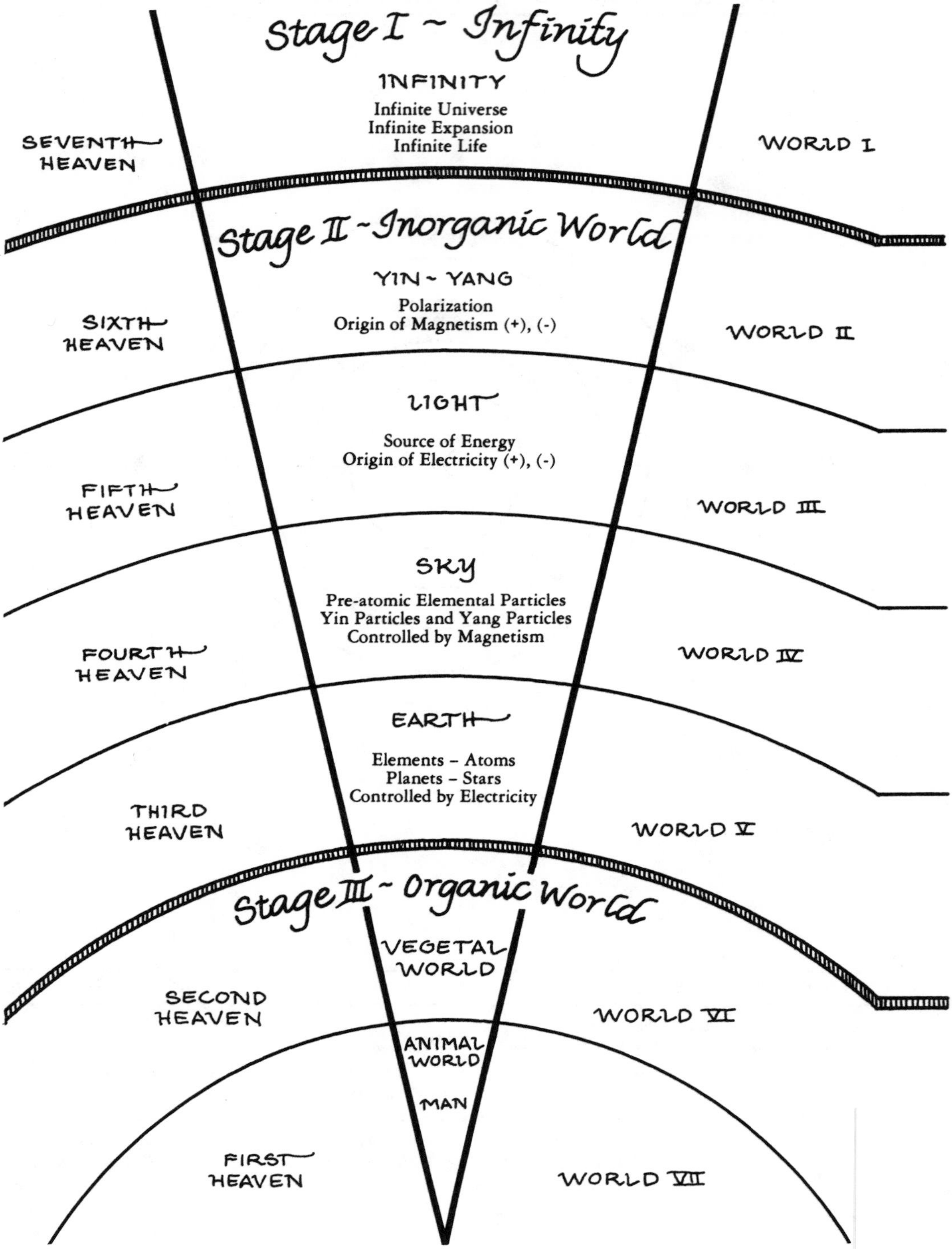

Stage I ~ Infinity

INFINITY

Infinite Universe
Infinite Expansion
Infinite Life

SEVENTH HEAVEN

WORLD I

Stage II ~ Inorganic World

YIN ~ YANG

Polarization
Origin of Magnetism (+), (-)

SIXTH HEAVEN

WORLD II

LIGHT

Source of Energy
Origin of Electricity (+), (-)

FIFTH HEAVEN

WORLD III

SKY

Pre-atomic Elemental Particles
Yin Particles and Yang Particles
Controlled by Magnetism

FOURTH HEAVEN

WORLD IV

EARTH

Elements – Atoms
Planets – Stars
Controlled by Electricity

THIRD HEAVEN

WORLD V

Stage III ~ Organic World

VEGETAL WORLD

SECOND HEAVEN

WORLD VI

ANIMAL WORLD

MAN

FIRST HEAVEN

WORLD VII

This diagram is a section of the logarithmic spiral which shows the continuity of the world of Infinity with the relative worlds. The first Six Heavens are part of the Seventh Heaven (Infinity).

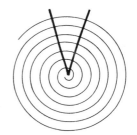

First Stage of Life: Infinity

Other names for World I are: Infinite Life, the Absolute, Oneness, God, the Almighty, the Tao, Highest Will, Supreme Judgment, Infinite Cyclotron, etc.

Second Stage of Life: Inorganic World

This is the boundary between the infinite world and the relative, finite worlds beyond which all analytical, mechanical and statistical science cannot go. Beyond here all tele-microscopic investigation is invalid.

World II is the foundation of the relative world. Yin is the origin of expansion and Yang, the origin of contraction.

This Stage of the inorganic world has been considered as the realm of Death. In reality, this Stage is the origin of biological life.

World III is the world of space and time, centrifugal force and centripetal force, dilation and compression, silence and sound, cold and heat, darkness and light.

World IV is the world of elemental particles, such as the electron and the proton and all the sub-atomic particles from which these are derived. All sub-atomic particles may be divided into yin particles and yang particles.

World V is the world of billions and billions of galaxies each containing millions and millions of solar systems. The theory of universal gravity is a misunderstanding of World V. The theory of relativity holds only for Worlds V, VI, and VII.

Viruses are found at this boundary between the inorganic and organic worlds.

Third Stage of Life: Organic World

The Constitution of the Universe, The Infinite World

1. The domain of life is made up of six levels: Human [animal]; Vegetal; Earth; Sky; Light; Infinity.

2. Each level is dependent on every other. All levels interface, just as certain objects lock into one another. The highest level is the Infinite. The Infinite is, therefore and by definition, without limits.

3. The levels pertaining to the finite world are not one-dimensional in form, but spherical, unfolding as a spiral. Yet in regard to the infinite world we are unable to qualify it either as spherical or rectangular, since the Infinite is without any form whatsoever.

4. The world that encompasses one or various other "worlds" penetrates to the most remote corners of those smaller worlds, while the latter occupy only part of those worlds greater than themselves.

5. Contiguous levels are always antagonistic according to the Order of the Universe. For example, movable and immovable, human and vegetal, Earth and sky, light and darkness, vegetal and Earth, etc.

6. Each level contains many antagonisms, oppositions, and contrarieties:

> *In the Human World:* man and woman, governors and governed, worker and capitalist, work and rest, love and hate, blood and tears, war and peace, happiness and misfortune, sickness and health, life and death, head and feet, hollow organs [lungs, stomach, intestines, bladder] and packed organs [heart, liver, kidneys, spleen, pancreas], bone and flesh, white and red corpuscles, nerves and muscles, sympathetic and parasympathetic nervous systems, tension and relaxation, spirit and body.

In the Vegetal World: grass and tree, trunk and branch, branch and leaf, flower and seed (or fruit), cell and organ, germ and soma cells, nucleus and cytoplasm, nucleolus and mitochondrion, individual and life as a whole.

In the Earth World: mountain and river, land and sea, air and earth, polar and tropical regions, hot and cold, day and night, surface and center of Earth.

In the Sky World: centrifugal and centripetal force, solid and gaseous.

In the Light World: visible and invisible radiation, hot and cold rays, dynamic, stimulating rays (yellow, orange, red) and static, calming rays (green, blue, indigo, violet), visible and ultra-violet radiation, infrared and visible radiation.

In summary, at each stage our analysis presents us with a number of antagonisms, oppositions, and dialectics. An overall synthesis, on the other hand, will show us one single antagonism, that is, the finite versus the infinite world, or the relative versus the absolute world. The more one continues on to the infinite world the smaller the relative world becomes until finally it disappears altogether.

The Order of the Universe

Having made our way up the River of Life we have at last discovered the Order of the Universe. It embraces all since it is the Order of infinite space and infinite time. The word "order" carries another meaning: command, directive, instruction. In China that is all summed up in one word: *Ming-Ling*. "Ming" means Heaven (yin) and "Ling," Earth (yang). Man is born between Heaven and Earth, and so must live according to the order of yin and yang. In this world all is subject to change; everything changes. Only the Order of the Universe remains unchanged. It's only natural that the finite world obey this Order of the Universe since the former arises from the latter. This Order is extremely simple yet it explains everything in the phenomenal world which can be understood in terms of yin and yang. [The concepts of yin and yang will be explained as this chapter proceeds. Ed.]

For example, a straight line is made up of innumerable points, each of which stands in opposition to its neighbors, that is, each point is to the right of the adjoining point on the left, and vice versa. When two things are in a relationship of "right-left" or "up-down," they infallibly attract and complement one another.

Although apparently contradictory, basically yin and yang complement one another; they get to know each other and join together. Although there are a number of words that approximate the meaning of yin and yang, I prefer yin and yang to these other expressions, such as more and less, positive and negative, masculine and feminine, good and evil, etc.

Even when the infinite and finite worlds are mutually antagonistic and contradictory, the one is part of the other, that is, we are dealing with the relationship between a part and the whole.

The Universe which manifests itself through the attraction and complementarity of yin and yang – man and the vegetal world, the vegetal world and Earth, Earth and Sky, Sky and Light – is the great harmony of the spheres. It is the Order of the Universe, the eternal

Order. Or better yet, for me it means the one and absolute Truth.

The dialectical method arrives only at an imperfect understanding of the Order of the Universe. It attempts to bring spiritualism and materialism together and harmonize them after the fashion of a mosaic.[24] It fails in this, despite its worthy intentions. One must necessarily take a stand in favor of one or the other position, much like a child who would hold that a human being originally comes from either the man or the woman.

The true source of man and woman, of materialism and spiritualism, and of their coming together (resolution of their duality) is the Universe, God, Nature, Life. The reason is that this Matrix has a built-in dualistic or inyological structure.[25] At any rate, all "-isms" are only partial visions of the Order of the Universe.

Imagine that the Universe is a cog wheel of infinite diameter.[26] Materialism may be thought of as the part that projects outward, the tooth, while spiritualism is more like the depression between the teeth. People who think dualistically or eclectically can only see the mountain or the valley; they can't take in the whole wheel. We haven't talked about the wheel's center, the axis, or about the motor. These we cannot know. Nor do we need to; those aspects we call the Infinite, the Absolute, God, Truth.

Continuing on with our image, we see that the first all-encompassing gearwheel (Infinity) interlocks with a second, called the world of Light. The two wheels revolve in reciprocal motion, in inverse order to each other (yin and yang). The diameter of this second gearwheel (Light) could amount to a million light years, but compared to the outer wheel, which is infinite, it would be considered infinitesimal. The second gearwheel is connected, in turn, to the third, the world of Sky, a world which doesn't display the great movement that we find in the second (Light), for it is yin. The third meshes with the fourth, the world of Earth, which is yang, and this, in turn, with the fifth, which is yin, the vegetal world. The sixth and smallest wheel is the world of man.

This image may help to describe how the Universe is constituted according to the inyological structure. It is my vision of the Universe, of the Unique Principle; it is my conception of the world.

Recently in reading Japanese mythology I was surprised to find a clear reference to the Unique Principle. In this account the god Ame-No-Minkamushi-No-Kami represents the Universe or the Infinite. Yin is represented by the god Takamimusubi, and yang by the god Kami-musubi. Moreover, it is stated in these writings that these three gods are all occult, that is, invisible.

It is amazing to find many similar myths in countries like China, India, and ancient Greece.

Democritus said: "The truth is that there exist only atoms and emptiness."[27] We meet the Order of the Universe in Genesis. Every classical work from ancient China teaches us how to understand the Order of the Universe and how to live in harmony with that Order. Everything called by the word *Dō* (*mitchi*) in Japan is an art or discipline based on the Order of the Universe. The word *Dō* can't be translated simply as "Way" or "Path"; it must include the meaning of commitment to the order of yin and yang, in other words, to the fundamental principle of the Universe.

The Japanese people place great importance on the word *gyo*. A proper understanding of this word requires that every action and thought concur with the Order of the Universe. For this reason those who live according to *gyo* must at all costs respect the Order of the Universe in every situation, insignificant as it might seem; for example, in the way we eat, the way we are seated in a room, the placement of our bed, the location of the bath, and so on. In all cases the inyological requirement always precludes any economic considerations.

The *haiku* is the shortest poem in the world. In only seventeen syllables it must express the Order of the Universe, Nature, infinite space and infinite time in terms of flowers, insects, the sound of water – in everything the eye perceives. One who has mastered the secret of this art is known as *haisei* (the saint of *haiku*). A saint is one who has tired of the pleasures and sorrows of this finite world, that is, one who knows the origin of this world, namely, the Order of the Universe. If Professor M. Planck had a real understanding of the word *Kendo* (the *Dō* of swordsmanship), he would be truly amazed.[28] So would he, too, if he knew that some people are honored with the title of *Tatsujin* in every class of *Dō*. For *Tatsujin* means that one has arrived at the mastery of his *Dō*. A curious aside: Up to the present time all Tatsujin were self-taught. The reason is that they had no choice but to practice *gyo* in order to learn their *Dō*.

The Unique Principle of yin-yang, which is a projection of the Order of the Universe, is very useful because of the following characteristics:

1. It provides structure and direction in all domains of life (spirit, body, discipline, technology, theory, practice, war, peace, etc.).

2. Everyone, old and young, can understand it and apply it in all aspects of life at any time and in any place.

3. It accepts all antagonisms, demonstrates their complementarities and mutual affinities, and includes everything. Consequently, even when someone adopts an exclusive and aggressive attitude towards us, we are capable of staying morally calm and taking responsibility for setting matters right.

4. It is found at the intuitive level in the myths of various ancient cultures, even though it may be only in an incomplete and partial form.

5. It is the eternal Order. There is absolutely no need to modify it. Once learned it will never be forgotten.

For a long time now I have set myself the challenge of explaining this eternal principle to Western peoples; my headquarters, a tiny garret in the heart of Paris, my resources, a life of poverty.

The task? To bring those who have been brainwashed by a materialistic and purely scientific way of thinking to a true understanding of the world, that is, to an appreciation of the Unique Principle. This little book is only a preface to the Order of the Universe. After finishing it I am resolved to write *The Order of Man, Health and Order, The Order of Politics, The Order of Economics, The Order of Agriculture,* and so on. In *The Order of Man* I will deal with every kind of problem facing human society; in *Health and Order,* with all types of illnesses; in *The Order of Politics,* with all the major political principles; in *The Order of Economics,* with the ethics of economics; in *The Order of Agriculture,* with life, blood, and the Earth. By reading these books you will come to understand how to apply the Unique Principle in practical ways.

* * *

When I wrote this book twelve years ago, I was very yin and shy. Therefore, I was reluctant to write the book, thinking that I would be making statements much too bold for such a young and unscholarly man. However, I am now sixty years old and am much more yang and less shy. Therefore, I am making some corrections and adding the following note:

1. All plants have chlorophyl, which makes them green. Take out the magnesium from the chlorophyl, replace it with iron, and the chlorophyl changes to hemoglobin, which is the essence of blood and, in turn, the essence of animals and man.

2. "Earth" means the elements of which it is made. The sun, moon, planets, stars, etc., are all made of elements.

3. "Sky" means the elemental particles of modern physics. (About fifteen have been found so far.)

4. "Light" means vibration or energy (E).

5. Light originates from the two antagonistic poles, which macrobiotics defines as yin (∇) and yang ($\triangle$), or, in other words, the relative world or Relativity.

6. Since the world of energy or vibration, the world of elemental particles (pre-atoms), the world of elements, the world of plants and the world of animals all come from the world of the two poles (yin and yang), antagonisms always exist, such as those between man and woman, life and death, young and old, right and wrong, beauty and ugliness, up and down, high and low, active and quiet, etc., in the world of man.

7. The origin of these two (yin and yang) is oneness, that is to say, Eternity, Infinity, the Absolute, Truth, Spirit, God, Love, Justice, Freedom, Happiness, the Tao, Nature, Nothingness, the Universe, etc.

8. Therefore, my original text – 1. animals, 2. plants, 3. Earth, 4. Sky, 5. Light, 6. Darkness – should be corrected to:

1. animals, 2. plants, 3. elements, 4. pre-atoms (particles),
5. vibration or energy, 6. the two poles of yin and yang,
or the principle of Relativity or change, 7. Eternity, Infinity, God.

The Twelve Theorems of the Unique Principle

We can summarize what we've said so far in the following way: The Unique Principle is a "polarizable monism," which means that the Universe is organized according to the inyological order, some examples of which are response, mutual correspondence, complementarity, and affinity. To put it another way, by means of the Unique Priniciple we arrive at a global view of all phenomena of life (which are only the natural development of that inyological order), thereby receiving a key that can unlock for us a life of health, happiness, and peace, and furthermore enable us to transform every misfortune into a celebration of life.

Another way of saying this is: The Unique Principle is a vision of the world which is based on the key idea of the unity of Spirit and matter. These are the twelve theorems of the Unique Principle:[29]

1. The Universe unfolds in accordance with the inyological order.

2. The inyological order operates continually and infinitely everywhere; the activity of yin and yang, mutually affecting one another, increases and decreases in endless cycles.

3. Yin refers to everything that exhibits a tendency toward centrifugal force, expanding, ascending, etc., while yang has to do with the tendency toward centripetal force, pressurizing, descending, etc. (For these reasons quiet, cold, and so on are manifestations of yin, while activity, heat, etc., are demonstrations of yang.)

4. Yin and yang are drawn to each other.

5. Every phenomenon is a complex bringing together of yin and yang in varying combinations and proportions.

6. Every phenomenon is but the coming together of yin and yang in dynamic equilibrium.

7. Nothing is absolute yin, nor is anything absolute and perfect yang. Everything is relative.

8. Nothing is neutral. The yin-yang polarization is incessant and universal.

9. The reciprocal attraction between things and beings is proportional to their inyological differences.

10. What are of like kind mutually repel each other. The force of the repulsion is equal inversely to the difference of the likeness.

11. At the extremes yin becomes yang and yang becomes yin.

12. All beings and things are charged with yang energy on the inside and with yin energy on the outside.

A Further Look at the Unique Principle

Now we will apply our Unique Principle to life. First, take a look at Map III (page 31) drawn by our Team of Life Explorers and notice the following points:

1. *Spirit Embraces All.* According to our map Spirit is Infinity itself and exists everywhere and at all times. With all the more reason then does Spirit encompass the relative world which is infinitesimal compared to the Infinite. This is because Spirit includes all.

2. *"I Think, Therefore I Am," or "I Am, Therefore I Think."* I think of something; therefore I exist. Is this assertion correct? According to our map Spirit is the infinite world. Spirit exists everywhere and at every moment. And so Spirit sees and thinks everything, every being past and future. The "I" that sees and thinks is the Infinite, the Universe, Nature, the Absolute itself. It's true that in the finite world there also exists an "i" that thinks and sees. But the former "I" is Infinity itself, not the "i" of man whose flesh is short-lived, existing as he does at this finite level.

3. *Chance Discoveries.* It seems that almost all inventions are always the work of chance: Watt's steam engine, Newton's law of universal attraction, Pasteur's innoculations, Galvani's electric current, Jenner's innoculation for smallpox, and so on.[30] In my opinion, those great men first reached the state of detachment and then, as their personal "egos" disappeared, were in direct contact with

45

the Infinite. And so their discoveries were the outcome not of chance, but of a state of inner readiness.[31]

When we think of something, most of the time we are only playing with knowledge, which is only a minute particle taken from that limited field of experience within the domain of the finite. But when we reach a state of detachment and free ourselves from all the "ego" emotions arising from our finite existence, we then find ourselves in the vast domain of the Infinite, the world of Spirit. Because this latter world encompasses all things, by entering it we enjoy a global view of reality that not only touches on every conceivable problem but also points the way toward some solutions. This state strongly resembles the experience of *Satori*, also known as "trance."[32]

4. *The Method of Dialogue.* Socrates and Plato regularly utilized the method of dialogue [the "Socratic method"]. That is because the use of yin and yang – in this case alternating questions and answers – is an excellent method of resolving problems, being in perfect alignment with the Order of the Universe. We can find this inyological structure in the body. Digestion is a good example of it. Saliva, as well as gastric and other digestive juices, are composed of a mixture of acids and alkalies. Other similar "dialectical" methods akin to the way of dialogue are used, for example, in chemical analysis, swordmaking, ice fabrication, the production of liquid air, nitrogen, etc. All of this, even for one unaware of it, is an unconscious imitation of the structure of the Order of the Universe.

5. *Free Will.* It would appear that the political order is based on freedom of will. But free will is synonymous with freedom of Spirit and Spirit is infinite. And so it is natural for the Spirit to be free. Still, many of the world's political systems have crumbled and disappeared without leaving a trace because their leaders mistakenly thought

that they could use their free will to maintain a position of power in the finite world. They forgot that in the relative world, which is finite, true freedom is not to be found.

6. *Is War Evil?* War is certainly evil in that it brings about the death of thousands of people. However, in the finite world opposing movements occur regularly in accord with the inyological order, so in that sense war is only a manifestation of yin and yang; in other words, it is an inevitable phenomenon of the finite world. In fact, without war there could be no peace. When yang meets yang they mutually repel each other (as the Tenth Theorem of the Unique Principle states) but later they fuse together because they are of the same nature. When yin meets yang they attract each other at first because they are of opposite natures, but later on they will struggle with each other indefinitely because they are opposites. Where you find good relationships there's no progress or creativity, but rather stagnation, rigidity, and hardening; on the other hand, where there is struggle, noble impulses and beautiful creations arise.

Weighing whether war is a good or evil depends on one's definition of good and evil. What is your point of view? War and peace, good and evil – all of these are of the relative, finite world. Therefore, they are all relative too. It depends on how you view the question. If we're looking at the infinite, absolute world, war is only one of the innumerable tiny waves produced within the finite world. If you focus on the crest of the wave, you think that war is okay, while if you're looking at the base of the wave, it would seem to be something bad. Some think that war is the origin of the development of culture. It's just a point of view taken from the relative, finite world.

7. *Is Life a Struggle?* It's just a fact that life is a struggle if we look at its ups and downs (the yin and yang of it) as a

kind of combat. Still this judgment comes out of the finite world and so lacks substance. All the better if struggle promotes strength in those who are too yin. At the same time we must not forget that all stimulation that goes beyond the balancing point can generate pessimism and despair, especially for those who are too yin.

8. *Causality and Moral Judgment*. Science systematizes what we call causality while ethics and philosophy determine moral judgment. Science is a discipline of "Sein" (Being), while philosophy and religion teach us "Sollen" (Duty, Responsibility). Science is a discipline of the relative world; moral judgment belongs to the infinite, absolute world. This is why science can never dictate to ethics. That the reverse sometimes happens is, however, only natural. Nevertheless our Unique Principle teaches us that the absolute, infinite world is supreme cause. From that point of view it is indisputable that the supreme cause is the source of moral judgment.

9. *Personality and the Soul*. If we define personality as the summation of all that goes to make up the individual – character, constitution, temperament, and so on – we could list a good number of elements that have the quality of Infinity about them, since the personality is only a combination of parts reflected from the infinite world on to the finite plane. Nevertheless, since all the elements of the personality originally arise at the level of the finite world, they are for that reason destined to disappear. The personality moves to the level of the Eternal by acquiring an originality that derives from its transformation into the great "I" which is of that other world belonging to the Spirit, the Infinite, the Absolute, Liberation. To put it another way, personality is of itself ephemeral. If the soul is the possession of the the individual, it will disappear with him since the physical body belongs to the finite world. But the soul is of the infinite world and therefore eternal, belonging, as it does, to the Absolute itself.

What is Life?

No one has ever been able to explain what life is in any compre-
hensible way. I consider life to be a passing phenomenon in our finite,
changing world. According to the map drawn by our Team of Life
Explorers, life is the inyological order that rules at the finite level.

And so nobody really knows what the origin of life is. According to
our map, it's clear that life comes from the infinite world. The dictum
"Every cell is engendered by another cell" is a truth of the finite world
and is to be validated only in the test tube. But where did the first cell
come from? "Omne vivum ex vivo" ("Every organism comes from
another organism") only holds true in the finite world. This Latin proposition is similar to the affirmation "Omne animal ex ovo" ("Every
animal comes from an egg") enunciated by William Harvey around
1650. Anyway, this is not a universal truth of Nature and the Universe.
Therefore, science cannot answer the question as to where the egg
comes from.

Spontaneous generation, seriously entertained at the beginning of
the seventeenth century, is not unlike our idea of God, as we saw above.
This theory was "destroyed" by some simple experiments like those of
Spallanzani, Gay-Lussac, and Pasteur.[33] These were valid experiments,
but they forgot to add "under such and such experimental conditions."
This unscientific way of looking at things may surprise us. But in spite
of this, their results are still taken for granted.

Recently a certain virus was discoverd that seriously challenges the
opponents of the theory of spontaneous generation.[34] In addition to
this, thanks to chemical research on proteins some scientists think that
it is possible to create organisms from inorganic substances in the
laboratory.

And so, without exception, all scientific theories pass away since
science only takes into consideration the beings and things of this finite
world. And so finite, too, is the duration of science.

The Principle that Unites Materialistic Science and Technology with Spiritual Philosophy and the Mystery Teachings

According to Map III the Unique Principle shows us that the Universe is made up of the material world of theories and technologies and the infinite world of the Spiritual, the Ideal, in accord with the inyological order, which manifests itself through correspondences, complementarities, and affinities.

We can understand, then, how these two worlds are the front and the back of one single world. We can translate them as body and Spirit.

Is Life Subject to Scientific Analysis?

According to Map III, the life of beings on the finite plane is the result of the development of the inyological Order of the Universe. On the other hand, that development is realized according to the law of the Fifth Theorem. ["Every phenomenon is a complex bringing together of yin and yang in varying combinations and proportions."] Also, we saw in the Second Theorem that inyological development is produced continually and infinitely everywhere, the activity of yin and yang mutually influencing one another, increasing and decreasing without end. Keeping these principles in mind we see that it is impossible to subject life to analysis, as if it were some dissectible body or chemical compound. Even if we were to succeed in analyzing life, the results would show up in mere abstractions and not in hard data.

What is Progress?

Progress means advancing in a certain direction which one has set for himself. Nevertheless, as long as one remains only in the domain of the finite world, advancement is not to be considered progress from the perspective of the Infinite. Sometimes, viewed from the absolute world, progress looks more like going backwards. Even as we advance, we are still only a geometric point on the map of Infinity. The same can be said of our regressions. Therefore, considered from the perspective of the Infinite, there is no observable difference in this world between advancing and retreating. Even supposing that what is happening seems to us to be real on-going progress, it may still end in failure, since progress is only the outcome of human observation, which is finite. However, if our "progress" is oriented in the direction of the infinite world, it will never suffer a "setback." It will be true progress, surpassing as it does this finite, material world. Outstanding inventions and discoveries have always been the creations of those who have succeeded in entering into the infinite world, that is, the world where the small "i" does not exist. At least, that is how I see it.

The Greater the Heat the Greater the Movement

This proposition holds true only at the finite level because heat and movement are found only on the material plane. The proposition is actually redundant.

The greater the movement – that is the greater the yang – the greater will be the yang of heat. Movement is the source of heat. Heat is *not* the source of movement. Both heat and movement are yang, a fact which indicates that they exist in the material (yang) world.[35] On the other hand, the source of the finite world is the Infinite; therefore the source of heat originates there. The origin of yang is yin, as the origin of the relative is the Absolute. This is a very important point. To put it another way, the infinite world, the domain of Spirit (or "non-ego"), is not a kingdom where Death rules, but rather a world emanating from Life, a world of Freedom, Equality. In the infinite realm only creation goes on, never the processes of death and decay. In fact, in this finite, material world there is absolutely no creation taking place. It can only occur at the infinite level.

How Have Things Arrived at their Present State?

This has always been considered to be a great enigma. Nevertheless, if you study Map III closely, you will be able to come up with the answer.[36]

Why Has Mankind Not Enjoyed Good Health Despite All the Progress Medicine Has Made?

Medical advances owe much to science. In order to understand life science first studies numerous phenomena and principles, especially in the fields of physics and chemistry, where research is limited to the material world. Since medicine has taken its principles from such technologies, it has as a result certainly realized some progress at the finite level. But in so doing it has moved a long way from the world of Spirit and from Life.

Darwinism[37]

The theory of evolution as proposed by Darwin has declined, as do all theories and scientific systems, sooner or later. In fact, that it is still alive at all is only because of the theory of heredity and the mystery of chromosomes.

If you take a look at Map III, you will clearly understand the mechanism of the theory of evolution. Though Darwin may have made his way up the path that leads to an understanding of how creation developed, his was really no more than a subjective commentary. He is like the person who describes the processes involved in a game of chess but forgets about the presence of the two players sitting there. If these players start a new game, the outcome will never be the same. All in all it's naive to think that there is only one theory of evolution as Darwin maintained.

There Is No Unity Without Obedience

If the Absolute, that is the Order of the Universe, is not obeyed, there can be no harmony. The present condition of the world says it, as clear as day. Ever since medieval religion which taught obedience declined, violent wars and lamentable struggles have intensified more and more upon the Earth. There is no way to keep an army disciplined without obedience.

The unity of the finite world (yang) is based on obedience to the infinite world. On finite levels a unity maintained by force or power is not lasting.

The Inyological Chart of Pythagoras[38]

1	2	3	4	5
infinite	even number	left	woman	dynamic
finite	odd number	right	man	static

	6	7	8	9
	curved line	darkness	bad	low
	straight line	light	good	high

Question: Can you correct this chart?[39]

The Characterological Types of Kretschmer[40]

Here are the four characterological types of Kretschmer:

1. *Cyclothymia on the Manic Side*: eager for pleasures, equally prone to getting worked up or calming down.

2. *Cyclothymia on the Depressive Side*: reactions flattened out, but slower; feels more comfortable leading an ordered life in which responsibilities are fewer.

3. *Schizothymia on the Manic Side*: two varieties – unstable and tenacious. The first is versatile, incoherent, noisy, alternately energetic or lazy, consistently undisciplined; the second type is hypersensitive, "spacy" and inclined toward mysticism.

4. *Schizothymia on the Depressive Side*: withdrawn from the world around him. Hard, intransigent, goes to extremes and has lost the capacity for compassion.

I wonder if Kretschmer knew the origin of these types. Anyone who ignores the importance of diet and the environment can't use this classification for the following reasons:

1. There are those who transcend these types and those who are exceptions.
2. Each one of these types can be transformed into another.
3. It's not possible to explain the "why's".
4. The relationship between these types and the Spirit is as yet unknown.
5. It is not known how to correct the defects of these types.
6. No suggestions are offered to improve the well-being of each type.

Is Justice the Same as Power?

Often it is assumed that power is justice and justice is power. This kind of justice exists only in the finite world. It seems that in the West the term "power" is linked to the words "justice" and "rights." An interesting phenomenon. In the Far East it's just the opposite. In his book Lao Tzu says:

The finest weapons can be the instruments of misfortune,
And thus contrary to Natural Law.
Those who possess the Tao turn away from them,
Evolved leaders occupy and honor the left;
Those who use weapons honor the right.[41]

However, in Justice there must be no weakness. Justice belongs to both Earth and Heaven; it is the Order of the Universe. Even though it is yin and without material power, when it is manifested in the finite (yang) world, it undoubtedly enjoys supreme dominion.

According to Michaelangelo's mural of the Last Judgment, the orientation of Paradise is to the left and that of Hell to the right.

The Whole and the Parts

"The parts make up the whole." This is the view of Totalism and derives from mechanical thinking. But if we say that "the whole precedes the parts," then we are guilty of dogmatic thinking. The idea that the whole and its parts coexist side by side is the democratic way of looking at the question. The relationship between the whole and its parts is usually misinterpreted. It may be understood, however, through a study of Map III. The whole is Infinity and the parts are of the relative, limited world. The usual way of thinking about it is that the so-called "whole and parts" are both situated in the relative world. And so their relationship is analogous to that which exists between Infinity and the relative world.[42]

The whole and the parts can be explained by using the image of a triangle. If a triangle represents the whole, such as a society, then a line or a point on the line represents the parts. Then if we divide the triangle by a horizontal line at half its height, we can split the triangle in two (upper part and lower part). The upper part is the leader class (yin) and the lower part is the controlled class (yang). Or we could say that the upper part consists of the capitalists and the lower part, of the laborers. We can go on to divide the upper part endlessly. Then the highest point will be the highest leader, such as the president of that society.

However, just lines and points do not make the triangle. It must have a power that binds it together. But even if there is a holding power, we do not have a whole triangle if there are no lines or parts.

This binding power is Infinity, or God. The three lines or points all come from Infinity. Therefore, in this relative world there exists the Order of the Universe. This Order I call "The Order of Man," "The Order of Society," "The Order of Politics," etc.

What Is Justice

Justice is the unfolding in this finite existence of inyological relativity, mutual response, complementarity, and causality; it means living in conformity with the Order of the Universe.

Time and Space

Space is of infinite expansion while Time is of infinite duration. Both are infinite, that is, both are synonymous with the infinite world, the spiritual and absolute domain. Space and Time are not two different things. Whoever would look at them as two is applying the standards of measurement of the physical body. The human organism is finite; consequently, when Space and Time are measured by the body's standards, they seem to be finite.[43]

Why do we view Space as three-dimensional? Because we see it through the body which is three-dimensional. Why do we understand Time as one-dimensional? Because we measure it by the commonly accepted one-dimensional standard. If we were to measure Space by the standards of the infinite Spirit (yin) instead of by those of the physical body (yang), we could then understand how it is infinite. We could also understand that there are really no dimensions of Time, neither past, present, nor future.

The past and the future are only directions, changes in relation to the body. If we switch directions the past becomes the future. Suppose we're traveling on a train from Paris to Moscow and that we are at this moment in Berlin. In this case Moscow represents the future for us. Now imagine we've received a telegram instructing us to return immediately to Paris. Then Moscow becomes the past and Paris becomes the future.

Don't forget that Space is the same as Time. I repeat: Why is Space viewed as three-dimensional? Because the human eye is structured for seeing in three-dimensions. But if we are structured for seeing with infinite vision, then everything in our vision *is* Infinity.

Matter, Mass, Energy

According to physics and chemistry, these three essential concepts are in themselves indestructible and unchanging. But they are only found in the relative world of finite matter. Who applies them to the infinite world? This would be quite a job for the laboratory. How can one who only believes in an ephemeral, finite world come to experience something of the Infinite?

The indestructibility and invariability of matter, mass, and energy are basic concepts of physics, but in my opinion these views are more infantile than they are scientific. It's as if a child, on receiving his monthly allowance from his parents, were to say, "The money in my pocket is indestructible and invariable," even though he knows that the money was the creation of his parents' efforts, not his.

Our finite world is constantly nurtured by the Creator, the infinite One. That is why matter, mass, and energy are inexhaustible on the physical level.

Moreover, when finite man in a finite world looks into finite matter, he thinks of his starting point (as does modern physics) as a limited, quantified world. What a mistake! Even when he should be thinking of matter, mass, and energy as arising from the infinite world, he obstinately continues to view them in images taken from the finite world, much in the way we are inclined to make an idol of God when He is not visible to us. This kind of representation is, in effect, nothing but a false god.[44]

Matter, mass, and energy are continuously being created out of the infinite world, the world of God. The three are actually one and the same. They are infinite and inexhaustible, like a huge, mighty current. Even though that current is in fact constantly changing, it seems unchanging because we experience only a very small part of it. And the proof of all this is that the fields of atomic science, quantum mechanics, and the first and second laws of thermodynamics all lie at a standstill.[45]

The Wonder of the Electron

The old physics thought that our world was composed of matter that could be seen with our eyes. They discovered about a hundred elements. Physicists thought that these elements were a never-changing reality. However, this dream was crushed in 1898. That was the year that radiation of active uranium was discovered.[46] Through this discovery scientists knew that the differences between the approximately one hundred elements were to be found in the constitution of those elements, which, incidentally, are made up of nothing but yin and yang electric particles. As a result of the discoveries made at this time, matter was supposedly made up of two kinds of particles, the electron and the proton. But nobody thought much about the origin or constitution of these electric particles. This is like the millionaire's son who always has money in his pocket but who doesn't know how hard his parents had to work to make the money.

This theory is childish because it presupposes two things, electricity and particles. This hypothesis gives rise to a lot of questions: How far apart are these particles? How do they work? Where do they come from, and so on? This hypothesis is an idol of God fashioned by the scientists. If scientists were to understand the reality of God, then science itself would take giant strides forward and reach Infinity.

In reality, there are no particles. Electricity is a limited glimpse of Infinity. The ultimate generator of electricity is the Absolute, the whole Universe, Infinity, God. Its production is unlimited. The concepts that matter (the atom) cannot be distintegrated or that mass never changes no longer hold, as recent experiments on the theory of energy have demonstrated.[47] We are reaching the end of a materialistic view of the Universe. However, so too will these theories of energy pass.

The First and Second Principles of Thermodynamics

According to von Mayer, "whatever the system employed to transform work into heat or heat into work, there exists a stable relation (J) between work (W) and the quantity of heat (Q)," and, in line with Carnot, "a heat-producing machine cannot function if the heat does not transfer from the direction of hot to cold."[48]

This is a great discovery. Nevertheless, since heat is found only in the finite world (yang), these principles hold only in the world of matter and energy. They cannot be applied in the infinite world. Often they are applied to the whole universe, those who do so maintaining that very soon the universe will freeze, turning into a world completely devoid of life. This way of thinking is a great error. For those who understand that the infinite world has created the finite, that line of reasoning is ridiculous. We can admit that the principles elucidated by von Mayer and Carnot are plausible; but still, if they don't shed light on the "why" of it, then they are only providing a glimpse into a field where vain imaginings, suppositions, and hypotheses are rampant.

The Dialectical Method

Hegel's dialectical method is well-known among modern methodologies.[49] It's a way of thinking about the world whose special merit lies in expressing the evolutionary development of nature and the march of history. In the vision of total evolution the struggle between contraries is expressed by "thesis," "antithesis," and "synthesis," each being a single moment in universal unfolding. Hegel, following the laws of logic, attempted to develop the idea of "negation" and the "negation of negation." Up to this point Hegel's dialectics resemble our Unique Principle. And that's why his method is found in the vanguard of modern-day thought.

Still, it seems to me that Hegel's way of thinking is egocentric, materialistic, and limited, given that his treatment of the antagonism between thesis and antithesis, or of negation and the negation of negation, is taken from a totally subjective point of view. What may be negation for one person can be turned into affirmation for somebody else. One is free to equate antagonism with contradiction. But this view will only lead to rigidity of conduct and to cruel and bloody acts, for example in matters concerning the relationship between rulers and subjects, men and women, rich and poor, life and death, good and evil. One who holds to such a categorical way of thinking believes that he is obliged for the sake of his own survival to enter into a struggle unto death as the way of his being in the world.

This rigidly categorical style appeared in Western thought with the arrival of Cartesian dualism and its offpsring – liberalism, individualism, evolutionism, democracy, etc. Nevertheless, Cartesian dualism never explains why there is contradiction between thesis and antithesis, between negation and the negation of negation.

Why is thesis negated by antithesis? Dialectics will not enjoy any credibility until it knows how to explain the second law of thermodynamics, above all, the most important part concerning evolutionary development. And so, why have thesis and antithesis appeared? What is thesis? What is antithesis? What is their origin? As long as these questions defy understanding dialectics will only be a way of thinking applicable to the finite, material world.

It has been suggested that the idea of Totality arose as a remedy for eliminating the defects of the dialectical method, to develop and complete it. Still, the method is lacking. At times the concept of Totality may emphasize antagonism through such terms as "opposition, contradiction, and negation"; at other times the concept may stress the aspects of "harmony and affirmation." Another possibility might be to consider "antagonism" as just a branch of Totality. But all these attempts to bring the idea of Totality to some form of unity still occur only at the finite level. As a result, we still don't know why the idea of Totality "ignores," so to speak, the function and workings of Creation.

Ideally what would complete that Totality is the Unique Principle or the concept of the infinite world, but not an ontology that would derive evolutionary development from Being, nor an evolutionary theory that would advance itself as the source of Being. In fact, it is the Unique Principle that demonstrates how Being *is* Creation, the Ideal, Life itself.

The most important challenge philosophy must meet is the understanding of how the *One* brings forth the *Many*. This question has not been settled either by Hegel's Dialectics or by the idea of Totality. Some day, when time permits, I would like to write an entire book on the subject.[50]

Conclusion

Our conception of the Universe needs to rest on a great principle. Such a principle must not only be valid for the finite world, but must be applicable to both the finite and infinite realms. Otherwise, it will not be a principle that allows for unification of all domains and which demonstrates the identity of matter and Spirit. Our conception of the Universe must clearly explain the relationships between health and happiness, between the body and the environment, between Spirit and body, etc. At the same time, it should be a principle that allows for the elevation of man's daily existence to a higher level, one that is marked by a healthy, happy, peaceful, free, and ideal way of life.

Again, I say: our conception of the Universe must orient us toward an unshakeable state of health and happiness. This view must be more than conceptual. Concepts are not real life. They are only photographs. The expression "conception of the world" is far removed from what I want to convey. My thought is inadequately translated by the expressions commonly used in Western tongues: "Conception of the World," "Conception du monde," "Weltanschauung," etc. My preference is "The Order of the Universe," "The Structure of the Universe," or "The Constitution of the Universe."[51]

However we say it, the Order of the Universe must be within the reach of all people and be easily understood by all. We must also be able to grasp it as one great overview of the structure and workings of the whole Universe. And finally, it must be applicable to our daily lives in a practical way. Regardless of how brilliant our theories may be, they will be useless and of no value whatsoever when it comes to curing illnesses.

Perhaps there are those who would think of our conception of the Universe as deriving from the Unique Principle to be somewhat infantile. If by "infantile" they are referring to the simplicity of a child, then it's true that the Unique Principle fits the description because its structure is made up of two elements only: yin and yang. It's as simple as a compass, but very practical and useful.

More than one hundred thousand people who have been helped simply by following the macrobiotic diet can testify to the benefits of the Unique Principle at the physiological level. In spite of this record, there are still an enormous number of recalcitrant souls who are unaware of the efficacy of macrobiotics. I wish I knew how to convince them.

Epilogue I

[This section, written in 1961, is a summation and update of *The Order of the Universe.* I recommend to the reader a rather careful study of it, keeping a finger on Map IV, page 32. Throughout Epilogues I and II bracketed, italicized guideposts have been provided to assist the reader in following Ohsawa as he drives us along some rather winding roads. Ed.]

What is life?

Life. Everyone knows life. Yet no one knows it. That's life.

Life follows three stages of development:

The First Stage is known as infinite expansion. It is the world that has no beginning and no end.

The Second Stage of Life is the spiral. Infinite expansion begins to polarize itself in Space and Time as a result of centrifugal force. The spiral is produced when the branches of polarization intersect and collide. The first circle of the spiral has two poles: yin and yang. In the second circle energy is produced. And in the third circle the elemental particles appear, giving rise to atoms, while these in turn through a process of compacting become the stars. That's how the first solar system was born and how millions of solar systems were created in a constantly expanding movement. This is the world of matter, the inorganic world.

The Third Stage of Life begins at a given place and moment in the world of matter. This is the organic world, a very small part of which is transformed into living beings. This happens naturally by spontaneous generation.

But now I don't have the time needed to explain this in scientific detail. I'll have to do it some other way.

In the infinite world there is no specialization.

[The Three Stages of Life and their corresponding Heavens and Worlds may be found on the left and right margins of Map IV, page 32:

Stage 1. Infinite expansion (Seventh Heaven = World I).
Stage 2. Inorganic life (Sixth Heaven through Third = Worlds II through V).
Stage 3. Organic life (Second and First Heavens = Worlds VI and VII).

The two paragraphs on memory which follow apply to the First Stage of Life, that is, World I. Ed.]

Why do we have memory, thought, will? Or how is it we dream of an ideal, of perfect health, of supreme justice?[52] Because we were born from an all-powerful and all-knowing Matrix, a fact which explains the infinite nature of memory. Our memory may not be able to describe in clear detail events prior to our early infancy, but it cannot be denied that such memory existed even before infancy. The existence of a memory that is prior to all beginnings and subsequent to all endings cannot be placed in doubt. What we call memory is essentially the big "I."

But why is memory hazy prior to birth? Because World I is absolute, infinite, and undifferentiated; consequently, it is beyond the awareness of our five senses. For the same reason, we are not able to predict the future.

[We now move quickly through the Second and Third Stages of life: Worlds II through V, and Worlds VI and VII, respectively. Ed.]

The Second Stage is the world of matter, the world of innumerable galaxies. It is the finite, relative, ephemeral world. Everything that exists in that world has a beginning and an end, a back and a front. There, all is dynamic and changing. There are no feelings in the world of matter, transition, and changeability. It is the inorganic world.

And of that inorganic world is born the world we call organic. And there in that domain of dream and illusion appear living beings, one part of which is humanity.

Only those human beings who have discovered the Infinite, that is, the Substance of life or the Matrix of the small "i," namely, those who belong to the infinite world, can realize their identity with Omniscience and Omnipotence. This state is known as "Satori," "Will," "Faith," or "Ecstasy."[53]

This is the meaning of life and of the Three Stages of Life. Those who haven't received this gift experience life as meaningless, often when they reach their forties. And at times some commit suicide as did Eastman, Hemingway, and others.

Such despair in the face of life is an example of how Order triumphs as an inevitable law of the Universe. This Order *is* Life itself.

Those who haven't been taught from an early age to bring order into their daily lives are incapable of putting their things and affairs in order if left to their own devices. And so their rooms, drawers, and heads are in hopeless disarray.

In summary, the Three Stages of life are:

1. Infinite expansion (World without beginning or end);
2. The spiral (the polarization of yin and yang), that is, the world of inorganic beings;
3. Organic beings (appearance of living beings), that is, the world of life.

The Third Stage of Life is what we know as our daily existence in this world. The Second Stage is the world of Death. So Death is the mother of Life. Life is a passage by which living beings are liberated from the finite world to enter into the First World (the Infinite, God), beginning at the human level, ascending through the animal and vegetal worlds, then on through the worlds of stars and elements, elemental particles, energy, the two poles of yin and yang, returning finally to the infinite world.

We call that First World: Brahman, Atman, God, Spirit, Amida, Tai-Chi (Tai-Kyoku), Father, the Infinite, Nothingness, Emptiness, etc.[54]

Stages II and III are characterized by changeability and uncertainty; they are the stuff of everyday life, passing worlds filled with illusion.

The First Stage, infinite expansion without beginning or end, penetrates into Stages II and III where it is given names like the Holy Spirit, the Tao, Yin-Yang, Dharma, etc.

One who in the Third Stage of Life teaches the Tao and the Dharma, offering the gift of peace to all people, is called sangha, son, saint, etc.

And so that is how we can grasp the true meaning of the Holy Trinity (Father, Son, and Holy Spirit), or of the Three-fold Treasure (the Buddha, the Dharma, and the Sangha).[55]

Many miraculous cures, many experiences of renewed body and spirit obtained through the macrobiotic medicine of the Orient show the superiority of this philosophy of the Far East in explaining the Three Stages of Life.

In the West there exists only one name for this First World: God.

The Second Stage is only an infinitesimal part of World I. It's like a geometrical point. Nevertheless, in this world we find innumerable galaxies. And each galaxy contains so many solar systems as to be almost beyond counting. Our Earth is just a planet of a single solar system. On only one small part of a small Earth live millions and millions of people. The Earth is a world infinitesimally small, like a grain of dust in a galaxy, but to man's vision it seems enormous.

It would seem to me that Western man has no idea whatsoever of the infinite dimension of World I. To speak of its immensity only inspires fear. Still, for the Oriental that vast world is cause for joy.

Men of science and philosophy apply themselves to the study of Stages II and III without taking into account the First Stage, the infinite world. They don't understand at all that the Universe is infinite; that's why for them Infinity is matter for analysis.

They take for their god the king of this finite world, be it a dictator or one who is endowed with brilliance, wealth, violence and power.

In the Orient the Tao is God, the Order of the Universe, the Dharma.

It's peculiar, but in the philosophical and scientific worlds of the West we find no explanation for the existence of Infinity, the Absolute, God.

Christianity confuses the First Stage, the infinite world, with the Second and Third Stages, which are relative. God is personalized. He is given names and even clothes. He ends up becoming a sounding board for peoples' whims and desires. Jacques Maritain affirms that the relationship between God and man is like a one-way street.[56] By this he means that God cannot be expected to wait upon our demands. Even though in the West there are a few who think about the infinite universe, they also tend to exhibit a certain kind of religiosity that can only express itself through celebrating rituals and building churches.

Freud, dominated by fear and obsessed with guilt, considered that
First, infinite World to be a dark abyss. It seems to me that Reich had a
glimpse of it, but he died a tragic death.[57]

Science is the illegitimate daughter of desire, which dominates the
investigation of Infinity, the Absolute, Eternity, in a relative, finite, and
ephemeral world. We might say that such desire is the product of a
nostalgia for the infinite world. I think that the efforts scientists make
in that direction are irrational, impossible, and futile. This idea creates
more and more catastrophes the more it develops.[58] Bertrand Russell
deplored our civilization, saying that we live in an insane world. Henri
Bergson wrote: "Intelligence is characterized by a natural incomprehen-
sion of life."[59]

Medicine is only a subscience which tries desperately to suppress the
fear that arises from not knowing our place in the First, infinite World.
It responds to illness with a frenetic attack on the symptoms, but without looking into its fundamental cause. Even when all the symptoms
are produced by man himself and when, as a result, one can only wait
for things to get better of themselves, medicine only looks to the super-
ficial causes, to which it assigns the responsibility for illness, and then
tries to exterminate them. It's much like the action of an ugly man who
tries with one blow to shatter the mirror that reflects his ugliness.

In my opinion science is the god of our times. All the more reason
we must seek the true God, the Infinite, the Absolute, the Empty – in
short, the Unique Principle, which manifests in the relative world.

Generally speaking, the oriental methodology of analysis is superior
to that of the West, but that is because Westerners are very nearsighted
or totally color-blind from the spiritual point of view.

The surprising advances of Western technology come, in my opinion, from its arrogance and baseness: "The bigger the back, the bigger
the front."

On the other hand, Orientals have the tendency to seek salvation
through faith and their creative artistic powers. Faith for them is a
state of soul in which one places confidence totally in the infinite, all-
present, all-knowing, and all-powerful world. Their artistic power
unfolds in their ability to hold a harmonious, global perspective in
regard to all things and beings, and to express this reality in an artistic

way. This in turn comes from their intimacy with the infinite world and its fundamental laws of yin and yang as found in the relative world.

If we can bring the East and the West together, each will derive great benefits from the union.

In Japan for some time now one hears this expression: "Japanese spirit and Western technologies." Take as your working principle the greatest force of action along with supreme judgment.[60] Conquer arrogance with humility. Let flexibility always overcome your rigidity.

I'll add a note:

If you don't understand my teachings on astronomy and on the negation of universal gravity and of the binding power of atoms, then you have only the lowest level of judgment (mechanical judgment).[61]

One who lives at this level takes life from a slave's point of view. He's only a puppet in a tragedy played out by those who live their lives in blind faith.

In our times most people live out their lives at this level. A bare handful of leaders possess the second level of judgment (sensory) as their highest attainment.

Even among religious and social reformers you will often find persons who are at this low level. Some of them use these occupations for the enjoyment and sale of pleasure.

A certain Mr. E. who came to Japan to learn macrobiotics said at a reception given in his honor: "In Japan one often meets a number of Japanese who imitate Westerners. You are just like Europeans. Why do you practice macrobiotics only in your own families instead of spreading these extraordinary teachings of the Unique Principle to the whole world? As if you were Europeans . . . "

I was shocked. But he's right. There seems to be no difference between Japan and the West. People only differ at the level of their judgment.

Epilogue II (6/20/61)

Since the First World is infinite, all that is infinite participates in it: infinite freedom, infinite happiness, infinite justice. . . .

All that exists in Stages II and III of the relative worlds is finite: finite freedom, finite happiness . . . That is, everything there is slavery, misfortune, disorder. . . .

The First World is the world of infinite, centrifugal force. The relative worlds are of infinite centripetal force. They are the domains of those who believe in the power of wealth, knowledge, violence and domination.

The free man who is attached to nothing is a citizen of the First, infinite World.

Ah! What greatness, what peace, what joy flow out from the world of infinite centrifugal force!

Notes

Journey Up the River of Life

1. Newton's three axioms or Laws of Motion are: "Law I: Every body continues in its state of rest, or of uniform motion in a right line, unless it is compelled to change that state by forces impressed upon it. Law II: The change of motion is proportional to the motive force impressed; and is made in the direction of the right line in which that force is impressed. Law III: To every action there is always opposed an equal reaction; or, the mutual actions of two bodies upon each other are always equal, and directed to contrary parts." Sir Isaac Newton, *Mathematical Principles of Natural Philosophy,* from *Great Books of the Western World,* Robert Maynard Hutchins, Editor in Chief, Encyclopedia Britannica, Inc., 1952.

2. Ohsawa's note to the 1958 edition of *The Order of the Universe* reads: "What I have called 'Sky' refers to pre-atomic elements. In current terminology it refers to elemental particles. It comes from an energy wave. You know that this wave arises from two antagonistic poles (centrifugal and centripetal forces). And the world of these two poles gives rise to energy, the elemental particle, the elements, the vegetal and animal and human realms. Therefore it is completely natural for life and nature to possess a dialectical structure. Nevertheless, the world of these two poles is only a part of the absolute, infinite, and eternal universe."

3. For Aristotle (4th cent. B.C.) the four basic elements of the physical world were designated as Earth, Water, Air, and Fire. Ohsawa accommodates himself to this scheme by a slight adjustment of terminology: Earth, which is composed of soil and water (Water), supports vegetal and (therefore) animal and human life. Earth, in turn, is supported by Sky (Aristotle's Air), although it must be remembered that by "Sky" Ohsawa means (in modern-day terminology) the elemental particles, as pointed out in the previous note. Finally, by way of Light (Aristotle's Fire) we arrive at the ultimate physical source of life, the primary energy field. Beyond this, of course, the great principle of yin and yang comes into view. It is the door through which the infinite world manifests to the physical plane.

   The account of the universe given by Aristotle's predecessor, Anaximander of Miletus (6th cent. B.C.) is strikingly similar to Ohsawa's: According to Anaximander, the cosmos "developed out of the *apeiron,* something both infinite and indefinite (without distinguishable qualities). Within this *apeiron* something

69

arose to produce the opposites of hot and cold. These at once began to struggle with each other and produced the cosmos." *The New Encyclopedia Britannica,* 1982 edition, Vol. 14, p. 250b.

4. In demonstrating the existence of Spirit Ohsawa takes as his point of departure the uncertainty principle of modern quantum mechanics, which holds that the precise location of a given electron in time and space cannot be predictably determined. So we cannot say what it is that moves or energizes the electron, a primary building block of matter. For man, however, it is certain that thoughts and dreams exist. For Ohsawa these "realities" can only come from Spirit. Spirit may be beyond the grasp of our understanding, but our thoughts demonstrate its existence, like the Zen image of the finger pointing to the moon. Later on Ohsawa will allude to the possibility of direct access to Spirit through the experience of *Satori.*

Ohsawa's compatriot D. T. Suzuki holds a similar view: *"'Cogito ergo sum'* is Descartes' pronouncement and, I understand, modern philosophy in Europe starts from this. But in fact the opposite proposition is just as true: *'Sum ergo cogito.'* Because being is thinking and thinking is being. When a man declares, 'I am,' he is already thinking. He cannot assert his existence unless he goes through the process of thinking. Thinking precedes being. But without being, how can a man begin thinking? Being must precede thinking. Without the eggs there are no chickens and without the chickens there are no eggs. . . . " ("The Oriental Way of Thinking," *The Essentials of Zen Buddhism,* E.P. Dutton & Co., 1962). Suzuki goes on from here to give this argument a decidedly Zen twist.

Recently, in reading a biography of the Danish quantum physicist, Niels Bohr, I was surprised to find the young Bohr (a contemporary of Ohsawa) struggling with the same questions Ohsawa is asking himself in this chapter. Bohr was influenced in his thinking by the following passage from Poul Martin Moller's *Tale of a Danish Student*: "How could then any thought arise, since it must have existed before it is produced? When you write a sentence, you must have it in your head before you write it; but before you have it in your head, you must have thought, otherwise how could you know that a sentence can be produced? And before you think it, you must have had an idea of it, otherwise how could it have occurred to you to think it? And so it goes on to infinity, and this infinity is enclosed in an instant." From Ruth Moore, *Niels Bohrs,* Alfred A. Knopf, 1966.

5. Ohsawa is probably referring here (and later on in this chapter) to Chuang-Tzu (the early Taoist sage) who had this now famous dream: "Once Chuang Chou dreamt he was a butterfly, a butterfly flitting and fluttering around, happy with himself and doing as he pleased. He didn't know he was Chuang Chou. Suddenly he woke up and there he was, solid and unmistakable Chuang Chou. But he didn't know if he was Chuang Chou who had dreamt he was a butterfly, or a butterfly dreaming he was Chuang Chou. Between Chuang Chou and a butterfly

there must be *some* distinction! This is called the Transformation of Things." Translation by Burton Watson: *The Complete Works of Chuang Tzu,* New York: Columbia University Press, 1968.

6. For further details and background on Ohsawa's life see Ron Kotszch's *Macrobiotics, Yesterday and Today,* Japan Publications, 1985.

7. I was unable to obtain any information about this film other than what is given by Ohsawa. Perhaps one of our readers can supply it.

8. Ohsawa studied and was much impressed by Lucien Levy-Bruhl's studies on the primitive mentality. Ohsawa's own book on the subject remains to be translated. Levy-Bruhl's work spanned six volumes and twenty-seven years (1910– 1937). His thought is best summed up in the now well-known expression *participation mystique.* "Levy-Bruhl wished to demonstrate, through the universality of some primitive aspects of mentality, the unity of the human mind in space and time. From the fact of belonging to an archaic or a modern culture, the mind may have a different orientation, but it stays the same; and always, to varying degrees, in its every resource, participation is at work." Lucien Levy-Bruhl, *The Notebooks on Primitive Mentality.* Quotation taken from the Preface by Maurice Leenhardt, Harper Torchbooks, 1975.

The Eternal World

9. Ohsawa might have listed any number of works from many cultures to make his point that all sacred literature speaks of the Order of the Universe. The *Koran,* for example, is conspicuous by its absence from Ohsawa's list. Some readers may not be familiar with the *Kojiki.* "The first written records in Japan are. the *Kojiki* and *Nihon Shoki,* chronicles compiled on court order and completed in 712 and 720 A.D., respectively. . . . The *Kojiki* and *Nihongi* are very important in understanding Japanese religion and the formation of Shinto. These works illustrate two all-important religious notions: first, the divine (or semi-divine) descent of Japan and her people, and, second, the proliferation of *kami* (spirits) intimately related to the land and her people." H. Byron Earhart, *Japanese Religion: Unity and Diversity,* Dickenson Publishing Co., Inc., 1974.

Herman Aihara has this to say about the Heart Sutra: "About five hundred years after Buddha's death, his teachings were compiled into thousands of volumes or books by his disciples. One of these is *Dai Han Nya Kyo (The Book of Supreme Judgment).* This book, consisting of six hundred volumes, was too large for most people to read, however. Therefore, it was revised and condensed into only two hundred and sixty-two words. This condensation is the *Han Nya*

Shin Gyo or *Maka Hannya Hara Mitta Shin Gyo,* which is one of the most important sutras of Buddhism and has been chanted often by all Buddhists. This sutra . . . is a teaching of what is Supreme Judgment, Infinity, or Oneness. I have never come across such a fine explanation of Supreme Judgment and Oneness in so short and concise a form as the *Han Nya Shin Gyo* except in George Ohsawa's *The Order of the Universe.*" Herman Aihara, transl., *The Supreme Judgment Taught by Buddha,* George Ohsawa Macrobiotic Foundation, Oroville, 1971.

10. Ohsawa is obviously referring here to a story that eventually became the well-known opera *Madame Butterfly* by Giacomo Puccini (premiered at La Scala, Milan, 17 February, 1904), although Puccini's Lt. Pinkerton was American, not Dutch. Puccini was inspired to write the opera after seeing David Belasco's play of the same title in London. Belasco, in turn, was indebted to an attorney-turned-writer by the name of John Luther Long, whose story, also of the same name, appeared in *Century Magazine* in 1897. Long claims he heard the story from his sister, the wife of a missionary stationed in Nagasaki, and that it was derived in part from a true incident. Information from William Ashbrook, *The Operas of Puccini,* Oxford University Press, 1968.

11. On February 5, 1597 Paul Miki, a Japanese convert and effective Jesuit preacher, and twenty-five companions, most of them fellow converts, were executed in the City of Nagasaki by being affixed to crosses and pierced with spears. Shogun Toyotomi Hideyoshi, at first open to the coming of Christian missionaries to Japan, later reversed his policy in an attempt to stem the growing tide of intrigue and subversion the Portuguese merchants and privateers used in their efforts to gain a political footing in competition for Japanese trade. Hideyoshi was successful. Christianity "disappeared" from Japan until the latter half of the nineteenth century. When Japan once more opened its doors to the missionaries, the latter were amazed to find pockets of Japanese Catholics who had maintained the practice of their faith in secret for over two hundred years without outside support. Rome's canonization of Miki and his companions as Catholic saints in 1862 was most timely. That same year the first Catholic Church was built in Yokohama, followed by a second erected in Nagasaki in 1864. This latter, known as the Oura Catholic Church, has to this day kept alive the memory of St. Paul Miki and companions.

12. Albert Einstein said of Max Planck (1858–1947), the "father" of modern quantum theory: "The state of mind which enables a man to do work of this kind is akin to that of the religious worshipper or the lover; the daily effort comes from no deliberate intention or program, but straight from the heart." And there is this quote from Planck himself taken from an interview: "Science cannot solve the ultimate mystery of nature. And that is because, in the last analysis, we ourselves are part of nature and, therefore, part of the mystery. But to my mind, the

more we progress with either, the more we are brought into harmony with all nature itself. And that is one of the great services of science to the individual." Ken Wilber, ed., *Quantum Questions,* Shambala Publications, Inc., 1984.

13. This is the "heart" not only of Buddhist teaching, but also of the Order of the Universe as taught by George Ohsawa. This teaching is the essence of the great body of Prajna-paramita literature which developed from the first century B.C. to about the tenth century A.D. in India and China. Most translations of the Heart Sutra (see Note #9) say it this way: "Form is Emptiness and Emptiness is Form," while Herman Aihara prefers this: "Matter is Infinity and Infinity is Matter." For more information on this literature see the works of the great English Buddhist scholar, Edward Conze, especially *Selected Sayings from the Perfection of Wisdom,* Prajna Press, 1978.

14. Max Planck would, I believe, agree with Ohsawa. Another quote from Planck's essay, "The Mystery of Our Being": " . . . It was not by any accident that the greatest thinkers of all ages were also deeply religious souls, even though they made no public show of their religious feeling. It is from the cooperation of the understanding with the will that the finest fruit of philosophy has arisen, namely, the ethical fruit. Science enhances the moral values of life because it furthers a love of truth and reverence – love of truth displaying itself in the constant endeavor to arrive at a more exact knowledge of the world of mind and matter around us, and reverence, because every advance in knowledge brings us face to face with the mystery of our own being." Ken Wilber, *Quantum Questions,* Shambala Publications, Inc., 1985.

15. One of the lines everyone remembers from the Star Wars films is "May the Force be with you!" Even in our popular culture the Infinite is ever lurking in the shadows.

16. That "only Nothing can bring forth Being" may be a scandal to Western peoples. This is because "Nothing" is taken in a nihilist sense, namely, as an empty void, leading to a meaningless and hopeless view of life. Only suicide or the pursuit of power and pleasure lie at the end of that road. This pessimism is not what Eastern thinkers and teachers mean by their emphasis on "Nothingness." For them the Absolute is Nothing because it is beyond our ability to conceptualize or to put into words. However, the experience of this Nothingness is available to us through various forms of meditation, active or passive, taught by the great spiritual leaders of all ages and cultures. A good example of a great Western teacher who reached God through his cultivation of "Nothingness" was St. John of the Cross, the sixteenth century Spanish Carmelite. For Juan de la Cruz the "todo" was to be found only in pursuit of the "nada." See also Note #54.

17. Like the dreamer who doesn't know that he is dreaming, directly experiencing, the inner observer being absent. Hence, no remembering. Similar to certain transcendent states described by the saints and mystics: "Nirvana," "Satori," "union with God," etc. In contrast to this state of "forgetting" or "not knowing," which Ohsawa describes in this chapter, there is the phenomenon, known as lucid dreaming, in which the dreamer is conscious that he is dreaming. Also, advanced Zen practitioners are able to maintain a high state of conscious alertness – being in the moment – no matter how "deep" the meditation. I suspect that Ohsawa would hold that conscious awareness of being in our dreams or meditations would indicate that these experiences are still of the relative world and therefore dualistic. In other words, if we *think* we are in the "other world" (Ohsawa's World I, the Absolute, God, etc.), we are not really in it, but still in this relative world. Only through Death or in this life through "Forgetting" can we truly enter that infinite world of the Beyond. For recent developments in the study of lucid dreaming at Stanford University Sleep Research Center, see Stephen LaBerge, Ph.D., *Lucid Dreaming,* Tarcher, 1985.

18. Here and below I have taken the liberty of using quotations from English literature to convey the sense of the sayings which Ohsawa obviously took from his own sources. The quotes are (in order): *Hamlet,* I, ii, 72; The *Bible,* The Book of Proverbs, 16:18; *Romeo and Juliet,* II, vi, 9. Several parallel sayings (taken from Lafcadio Hearn's *In Ghostly Japan,* Charles E. Tuttle Company, 1971) are: "Life is a lamp flame before a wind." "This world is only a resting place." "Pleasure is the seed of pain; pain is the seed of pleasure."

19. A frequent theme in the Gospels: "And if you have faith, everything you ask for in prayer you will receive." Matt. 21:22. "Ask and it will be given to you; search, and you will find; knock, and the door will be opened to you." Matt. 7:7.

20. From Francis Bacon and Percy Bysshe Shelley, respectively. And several more from Lafcadio Hearn: "Meeting is only the beginning of separation." "All that live must surely die; and all that meets will surely part."
     There is a gentle poignancy to Ohsawa's own expression of this feeling in his song, "Wakare No Uta" ("The Goodbye Song"). This song is sung at the traditional closing of the Aihara's annual summer camp in the Tahoe National Forest. It is almost impossible not to experience the transitory nature of life as the campers sing this song, hands clasped in wide circle around a flickering campfire, saying goodbye to one another in Japanese, Chinese, African, French, and English:

> Meeting is the beginning of separation,
> Separation is returning to the beginning,
> Therefore, the joy of meeting is ephemeral and sentimental,
> However, a joy in our memory is eternal.

Sayonara, Tsuai chen,
De sudania, Bon voyage,
Good luck, Good luck,
Mata aima shyo,
The land of memory is the land of mystery
And the land of eternity.
Adieu! Adieu! Adieu!

21. "Everything is always changing, passing away. True joy and freedom can be found only by returning to the cosmic Self or *Tai-Kyoku (le grande Moi)*, and by transcending the ego self or *le petit moi*." Ronald Kotzsch, *Macrobiotics, Yesterday and Today,* Japan Publications, 1985.

Maps Used by the Team of Life Explorers

22. According to information provided by Herman Aihara, the first three maps consisting of simple concentric circles were used prior to 1947. Around that time, following up on a student's suggestion, Ohsawa redesigned his map in spiralic form. Later on, about 1960, Ohsawa began using the section or "piece of pie" taken from the spiral, which appears in this book as Map IV. In preparing Map IV for publication in this edition of *The Order of the Universe* Herman Aihara added some refinements and clarifications. This final version appears in the text on page 32. This map will serve as an essential guide in following Ohsawa through the Conclusion, pages 61–68.

23. Ohsawa, following his rather simple conceptualizations (maps) of the Order of the Universe, lists only six levels here. But if we are referring to the definitive outline [see previous Note #22], we find that Ohsawa changed it from six to seven levels to allow a place for the Yin-Yang polarity which serves as the gate between the infinite and finite worlds. So after [5] "Light," we must add [6] "Yin-Yang," and push "Infinity" to the seventh level. As the reader will note, this is the arrangement followed in Map IV, as previously indicated.

The Order of the Universe

24. The world "spiritualism" may present some difficulties for the reader. Here it does not refer to the practices of "spiritualists" who claim to be in contact with spirits "from the other side," but rather to the "philosophical doctrine that all reality is in essence spiritual." (*Webster's New Twentieth Century Dictionary, Unabridged, 1968.*) Ohsawa uses it in opposition to "materialism." See Chapter II

where Ohsawa criticizes both materialists and spiritualists as being too one-sided, the former being nearsighted, the latter, blind. This dualistic conflict can only be resolved at the level of the Unique Principle by living according to the Order of the Universe.

25. "Inyological." Ohsawa, who was quite fond of neologisms, coined this hybrid to express the essence of his yin-yang philosophy. The prefix "inyo" is made up of the Japanese "in" or "yn" meaning yin, and "yo" meaning yang.

 yn   *yo*

The suffix "logical" comes of course from the Greek "legein" meaning to gather, to read, or to recount. "Inyological," therefore, refers to the reasoning behind, and the explanation of, the yin-yang principle.

26. With a little imagination this figure of the epicyclic gear train may give the reader a picture of what Ohsawa is describing:

Instead of two inner wheels, there would be for Ohsawa, five (working from the outside in): Light, Sky, Earth, vegetal, man. Light would be the largest of the inner wheels and man, the smallest. Each wheel moves in the direction opposite to its connecting neighbor. What is missing from this image is the second world of Ohsawa's Map IV, the world of yin and yang. Since the yin-yang principle influences *all* the worlds beneath it ("Light" through "man"), perhaps it would be inappropriate for it to be represented by a wheel that turns in only one direction.

27. Democritus (5th cent. B.C.) taught that "an infinite number of eternal and uncaused atoms . . . invisible, differing from one another only in shape, arrangement, position, and magnitude . . . move through infinite space, or the Void . . . which though incorporeal, is existent and therefore real. Atoms and the Void are for Democritus the two ultimate realities." *Encyclopedia Britannica,* vol. III, p. 460b. This, of course, is a dualistic position and I believe Ohsawa would critique it on that score. It is only a partial understanding of the Universe. Is Democritus confusing Space with Void, the same mistake made by our contemporary Space explorers (see "Introduction," pages 1–10)? The Void is "beyond"

Space. It is the Matrix of both Time and Space, and of all created "atoms." It is the Absolute, the Infinite, God, etc.

28. Ohsawa writes: " . . . If you are not in good health, you must study the theory of Judo that I am explaining here because all the *Dō* schools (Judo, the Art of Defense; Kendo, fencing; Ido, medicine; Syodo, writing; Kado, poetry, and so on) are only different ways to enter into the same world of Peace and Liberty." (From *The Book of Judo,* serialized in *Macromuse,* Fall 1983, Winter 1984, Spring 1984, Summer 1984.) According to Herman Aihara, Ohsawa was the one who introduced the concept and practice of *Dō* into Europe during the 20s.

29. There are some differences in the wording of the Twelve Theorems as they appear in other works by Ohsawa. For purposes of clarification and understanding, the following versions from *The Book of Judgment* (George Ohsawa Macrobiotic Foundation, 1980) and *Zen Macrobiotics* (Ohsawa Foundation, 1965) are given with the version of *Zen Macrobiotics* in brackets where it differs from that of *The Book of Judgment.*

 1. Yin and yang are the two poles of the infinite expansion.

 2. Yin and yang are produced infinitely and continuously [and forever] from the infinite pure expansion itself.

 3. Yin is centrifugal; yang is centripetal. Yin, centrifugal, produces expansion, lightness, cold, etc. Yang, centripetal, produces constriction, weight, heat, light, etc.

 4. Yin attracts yang; yang attracts yin.

 5. All [things and] phenomena are composed of yin and yang in different proportions.

 6. All [things and] phenomena are constantly changing their yin and yang components. Everything is restless.

 7. There is nothing completely yin or completely yang. All is relative.

 8. There is nothing neuter. There is always yin or yang in excess.

 9. Affinity or force of attraction between things is proportional to the difference of yin and yang in them.

 10. Yin repels [expels] yin; yang repels [expels] yang. The greater the difference, the weaker the repulsion. [Expulsion or attraction between two things yin or yang is in inverse proportion to the difference of their yin or yang force.]

 11. Yin produces yang; yang produces yin in the extremity.

 12. Everything is yang at its center and yin at its periphery (surface).

A Further Look at the Unique Principle

30. "The great breakthrough (in treating smallpox) came in England in 1796, when Edward Jenner performed his innoculation experiment with material from a postular cowpox lesion on the hand of a dairymaid. Within a few years cowpox material was distributed around the world . . . " *Encyclopedia Britannica,* vol. IX, p. 280b.

31. A recently published book corroborates Ohsawa's opinion. Reviewing Roy Rowan's *The Intuitive Manager* (Little, Brown, 1986), *Time* states that Rowan "celebrates what he calls the Eureka factor, the sudden, illuminating flash of judgment that actually guides many business leaders. Logic is only one part of the decision making, Rowan contends; it is often the daring, instinctual leap that can make all the difference. . . . A formidable enemy of intuition, according to Rowan, is 'analysis paralysis,' a condition caused by too much inquiry. 'Constantly accumulating new information . . . without giving the mind a chance to percolate and come to a conclusion intuitively can delay any important decision until the time for action expires,' he says. That is 'substituting study for courage.'" *Time,* April 21, 1986.

32. The following is from a Zen (Ch'an) Buddhist document of the 8th century A.D.: "An infinitesimally small space contains all the phenomena of the great thousand-world system. An instant of time includes all the times of past, present, and future. . . . One thing is everything, everything is one thing. Causal origination has no obstructions: inner truth is clear in each and every thing. Thus we know that however broad the cosmos, it can fit into an atom of dust without being cramped. However long past, present, and future are, they can be contained in a brief moment. Thus we can see through metal walls, observing that there is nothing to be measured; we can pass through stone walls without any obstruction. Thereby do the sages find inner truth and perfect their functioning. If inner truth did not let them be so, the sages would not have such power. Liberation is penetration through inner truth. Obstruction is due to blockage by sentiments. The wisdom of the universal eye can see things as they really are." J.C. Cleary, transl., *Zen Dawn,* Shambala, 1986.

33. Lazzaro Spallanzani (1729–1799), Italian physiologist, made important contributions in the field of microbiology and bodily functions. Joseph-Louis Gay-Lussac (1778–1850), French chemist and physicist, pioneered studies on the behavior of gases leading to the discovery that all gases expand by equal amounts for equal increments in temperature; he also worked toward improving techniques for analyzing organic compounds.

34. Although the discovery Ohsawa refers to here cannot be identified, Herman Aihara, one of Ohsawa's most prominent students, is of the opinion that viruses may arise spontaneously. This is based on the understanding, for example, that "the growth of the AIDS virus is not the cause, but the result of illness. Such viruses can only multiply when the immune system is already unhealthy. Also, in my opinion," Aihara continues, "and from a macrobiotic point of view, the AIDS virus is produced in our intestines when the foods we eat contain synthetic materials." Herman Aihara: "Herpes and AIDS – an Update," *Macrobiotics Today,* May 1986.

35. Here Ohsawa is using the "inyological" concepts of yin and yang analagously, the finite world being viewed as "yang," the infinite world as "yin." The source of the comparison is the truth Ohsawa expresses a few lines later, namely, that the "origin of yang is yin," *just as* the origin of the relative world is the absolute world.

36. This question along with Ohsawa's terse and cryptic response is, according to Herman Aihara, the key issue in macrobiotic inquiry. Human science for all its technology and sophistication has not been able to come up with answers to the most fundamental questions dealing with the origin of things. What is the origin of a virus, DNA, the human species, etc.? How did every *thing* come to be in the finite world? Ohsawa wants to the reader to consider this question for himself. It is the great macrobiotic *koan.*

37. See also Herman Aihara's views about Darwinism, page 89.

38. "Aristotle's table of the Pythagorean opposites is as follows:

Limited	Unlimited
Odd	Even
Unity	Plurality
Right	Left
Male	Female
At Rest	In Motion
Straight	Curved
Light	Darkness
Good	Evil
Square	Oblong

Encyclopedia Britannica, vol. VII [Micropaedia], p. 554.

39. Answer: "If the upper row is yin and the lower row is yang, numbers 2, 5, 8, and 9 must cross over from the upper side to the lower side." (Herman Aihara)

40. Ernst Kretschmer (1888–1964), a contemporary of Ohsawa (1893–1966), was a German psychiatrist who was interested in correlating certain body types with specific psychological states. His best known work, *Physique and Character,* went into its 20th edition in 1947 and so would possibly have been read by Ohsawa. Here Ohsawa excerpts the concepts of "cyclothymia," a condition characterized by mood swings and assigned by Kretschmer to the "pyknic" (yang) body type, and "schizothymia," a condition marked by the tendency to split character and introversion, matched to the "leptosomic" (yin) body type. Although Kretschmer is no longer in vogue in the field of psychology, I decided to include Ohsawa's critique anyway, since it applies equally well, in my opinion, to many current offerings in the psychological marketplace.

41. Of the many available translations of the *Tao Te Ching* I have selected a very recent one, R.L. Wing, *The Tao of Power,* Doubleday & Company, Inc., 1986.

42. What is commonly thought of as "the whole" is, considered from the point of view of the Order of the Universe, itself only a part, since it belongs, like its "parts," to the relative world. This may seem to be a mere analogy, but it has important consequences. For example, all "-isms" in the political order come from totalitarian thinking, a dictator, for example, proposing that his particular "-ism" is the answer to the world's problems. The same may be said of the fields of religion, medicine, psychology, and sociology, where totalistic views are played out, usually with consequent harm to individuals and society. All "-isms" are worthless when viewed in the light of the Infinite.

43. My understanding of Ohsawa's thought about Time and Space is as follows: In Map IV Time and Space are found in the Fifth Heaven and therefore definitely belong to the relative world. Space is yin and Time is yang. But, considered from the point of view of the Seventh Heaven, the absolute world, both Time and Space are without limit or definition. In other words, at that transcendental level the laws of the relative world (as, for example, in physics or biology) do not apply. In the Space of Eternity there is no "where" for us to go, because we are already everywhere. The same with Time. In the absolute world there is no before, after, or even "now."

44. If Ohsawa seems to be defying the law of conservation of energy and matter, it is not, in my opinion, out of sheer contrariness. This law, he would agree, is perfectly valid at the finite level. But I believe he is warning us that we must look to the source of this law, namely, the infinite, absolute world, or God. The price we pay for not doing this is illness, smallness of mind, and poverty of life. We cannot place limits on the bountifulness of an infinite resource. Nor is there room in this view for any pessimism whatsoever, even in the face of nuclear disasters or threats of biological annihilation.

45. Here is a summary of the laws of thermodynamics: "The most useful statement of the first law (of thermodynamics) is that the change in internal energy of a system is equal to the heat absorbed by the system less the work done by the system on its surroundings. In this statement, a distinction is made between heat flow and the transfer of all other kinds of energy. The second law . . . has to do with the nature of thermal energy (heat) and temperature. It reflects the experience that heat flows from a higher to a lower temperature but that it does not do the reverse. The second law is best formulated in terms of entropy (measure of disorder at the molecular and atomic levels)." *Encyclopedia Britannica,* vol. IX, [Micropaedia], p. 947b.

46. The year 1898 was the year Pierre and Marie Curie discovered radium. With the assistance of the chemist Eugene Demarcay, an expert with the spectroscope, they found in their most active specimen "a single line in the ultraviolet range which did not belong to the pattern of barium composing the bulk of the material, nor of the platinum of the wire by which he (Demarcay) drew his sparks, nor indeed to the pattern of any known element. On this evidence, on the basis of its radioactivity, of its partial separation from barium, and its single spectral line, the Curies announced their second new element at the very end of 1898, and for the great intensity of its rays they named it radium." Alfred Romer, *The Restless Atom,* Anchor Books, Doubleday & Company, 1960.

47. Ken Wilber echoes what I believe to be Ohsawa's intuition: " . . . All things are *not* ultimately made of subatomic particles; all things, including subatomic particles, are ultimately made of God. And the material realm, far from being the most fundamental, is the *least* fundamental: it has less Being than life, which has less Being than mind, which has less Being than soul, which has less Being than spirit. Physics is simply the study of the realm of least-Being." Ken Wilber, ed., *Quantum Questions,* Shambala Publications, Inc., 1984.

48. In 1844 Julius Robert von Mayer (1814–1878), a German physicist, "postulated that in a work-producing cycle the heat introduced must exceed the heat rejected by an amount proportional to the work." *Encyclopedia Britannica,* vol. 18, p. 291a.
   Nicholas Leonard Sadi Carnot (1796–1832), a French physicist, "set forth the theory of engine efficiency, now known as *Carnot's Principle,* which states that heat cannot pass from a colder to a warmer body; and that the efficiency of an engine depends upon the amount of heat it is able to utilize. This hypothesis has been expanded into the second law of thermodynamics." *Funk & Wagnall's Encyclopedia,* vol. 5, p. 1816.

49. George Wilhelm Friedrich Hegel (1770–1831), the great German Idealist, was a philosopher of extremely wide range and a most prolific writer. His

dialectics may be studied in depth in *Hegel's Science of Logic: Muirhead Library of Philosophy*, Muirhead Library of Philosophy, 1976, as well as in various anthologies and commentaries.

50. Ohsawa kept his promise in *Atomic Age and the Philosophy of the Far East*, (George Ohsawa Macrobiotic Foundation, 1977) and in the "Epilogue" in this book (page 67). *Atomic Age*, now out-of-print, is scheduled for a new edition in the near future.

Conclusion

51. Since Ohsawa often interchanges the words "world" and "universe," and in order to avoid confusion for the reader, I am limiting the use of "Universe" to the totality of both infinite and finite worlds. The word "world" will ordinarily be used to mean realm, level, domain, etc., except when qualified by the adjectives "infinite" or "absolute," in which case it will refer to Infinity or the Absolute, which for Ohsawa is all inclusive, therefore "Universe."

52. Supreme justice is a term Ohsawa uses to express the ideal of living in complete harmony with the Order of the Universe. For an elaboration of Ohsawa's teaching on the levels of judgment, see Note #60.

53. There are two ways to reach the First Stage of Life: the long way, by following the path back up the spiral through the Third Stage of Life, then up through the Second Stage, the inorganic world which is also the gate of Death. Or we may take the shorter path if we are lucky enough to experience *Satori*, ecstasy, (or whatever name you may call it), a gift freely received from God for which our spiritual practices and deeds of kindness and compassion are only the remotest preparation.

    Satori, a term borrowed from Zen Buddhism, means the direct experience of the infinite world achieved through meditation. A Buddhist scholar, Garma C.C. Chang, writes: " . . . Zen work consists of two main aspects, the 'View' and the 'Action,' and both are indispensable. A Zen proverb says: 'To gain a view, you should climb to the top of a mountain and look from there; to begin the journey [of Zen] you should go down to the bottom of the sea and from there start walking.' Although the edifice of Zen is supported by these two main pillars, the 'View' and the 'Action,' Zen teaching lays most of its stress on the former. . . . Zen Masters put all their emphasis on *Satori* and concentrate on bringing their disciples directly to it." *The Practice of Zen*, Harper and Row, 1959.

    Of course, all religious disciplines urge their followers toward such experiences, which is the same for all, though the names are different. Spanish mystics, for example, speak of "transforming union with God." For an in-depth treatment of "Satori" see Heinrich Dumoulin, *Zen Enlightenment,* Weatherhill, 1983.

54. Again, Ohsawa is teaching that it doesn't matter by what name the infinite world is called, whether in personalized or abstract form. The names given here are taken from both Western and Eastern traditions. That God can be expressed by the terms "Nothingness" or "Emptiness" may cause some trouble for Western believers, but is no problem for those steeped in oriental thinking.

Here is one view presented by a contemporary Japanese Zen master: " . . . Absolute being doesn't belong to the objective world. The absolute world embraces subject and object together. The human being, believing he belongs to the subjective side and standing in the small mind, observes absolute being as object. Actually, that absolute being cannot be an object. Shakyamuni (Buddha) said that absolute being has no color, no form, no voice and exists as nothingness or emptiness. Absolute being works as complete, perfect emptiness and embraces subject and object. If you want to see God or Buddha, you must manifest yourself as emptiness. At the moment you manifest your imperfect consciousness as nothingness, your imperfect consciousness becomes perfect and illuminated." Joshu Sasaki Roshi, *Buddha Is the Center of Gravity,* Lama Foundation, 1974.

55. "Sangha" is the brotherhood and sisterhood of believers in the Buddhist tradition. The "Dharma" is the great teaching of the Buddha. And so there is the Buddhist "Trinity" of Dharma, Buddha, and Sangha. The Dharma is the infinite world [World I]; the Buddha in his celestial body is the Way to Infinity and is found at Stage II [Worlds II through V] to teach and assist the seekers; the Sangha, the flesh-and-blood body of the Buddha's followers, is of Stage III [Worlds VI & VII]. Similarly, in Catholic theology the Father represents the infinite world; the Son in his glorified body, the Second intermediate Stage; and the Holy Spirit, the divine presence residing the Christian community, the Third Stage of Life.

56. Jacques Maritain (1882–1973), a native of France and a convert to Catholicism, was the leading exponent in his day of Thomism (the philosophy of Aristotle adapted to the principles of Catholic theology by the twelfth century genius, St. Thomas Aquinas). One of his major works, *The Degrees of Knowledge* (1937), might be considered to be a Catholic interpretation of the Order of the Universe. I do not know the source of the reference made by Ohsawa in the text.

57. Wilhelm Reich (1897–1957) had much in common with Ohsawa. An original and unorthodox thinker, Reich contributed much to the wholistic approach to health and happiness that has emerged in our day. Like Ohsawa, he was criticized and ostracized by the current establishment. Reich's training was as a psychiatrist (he was one of Freud's students), but he took off on a completely new track: the

relationship of illness and health to the energy cycles of the universe (to which energy Reich gave the name "orgone"). He was intrigued with the possibilities of capturing this life energy, especially in the healing of cancer. He constructed and marketed a box which, he claimed, accomplished that end. He was indicted by the FDA for this and ended his life in the Lewisburg Penitentiary, dying of a heart attack in 1957.

58. Ohsawa calls this kind of thinking "sentimentality." For a contemporary example of this kind of thinking see my "Introduction," page 7.

59. Bertrand Russell (1872–1970), the British philosopher, is known especially for his work in mathematical logic and for espousing humanitarian causes. Like Ohsawa, he was twice imprisoned (in 1918) for his pacifist views.

Henri Bergson (1859–1941), a French philosopher, was a major force in the war against scientific determininsm. One of his key contributions to modern philosophy was the concept of *elan vital,* which, Bergson postulated, lay behind all change, especially evolutionary development. Like Ohsawa, Bergson favored intuition over reason. Among those who attended his lectures at the College de France was Jacques Maritain. See Note #56.

60. Here and in the following paragraphs Ohsawa speaks of high and low levels of judgment. For those unfamiliar with Ohsawa's thought, here is a summary taken from *The Book of Judgment* (George Ohsawa Macrobiotic Foundation, 1980):

"Our happiness depends upon our judgment. Illness or health, intelligence or foolishness, piety or vice depend upon our judgment. Judgment develops upward toward perfection, in the way I show below, from one to seven.

1. Physical judgment (mechanical and blind judgment).
2. Sensorial judgment (pleasant and unpleasant).
3. Sentimental judgment (what is desirable and undesirable).
4. Conceptual judgment (intellectual, scientific).
5. Social judgment (social reason's judgment: morals and economy).
6. Judgment of thought and thinking power (justice and injustice).
7. Absolute and universal love that embraces everything and turns every antagonism into complementarism. (p. 97.)

61. Here Ohsawa is taking a "potshot" at commonly accepted views in regard to gravitation and the nature of the atom. In effect, Ohsawa teaches that our view of the universe is myopic. What we think of as gravity is actually the centripetal force pushing into the center of the solar system, resulting from the tremendous

centrifugal force of an expanding universe propelled by Infinity. In the same way, the constituents of atoms are "pushed together" by this awesome force, leading to the building blocks of all creation, both inorganic and organic. These views were later developed in *Atomic Age and the Philosophy of the Far East* (George Ohsawa Macrobiotic Foundation, 1977).

A similar view is given by Joshu Sasaki Roshi: "You have a center of gravity which is opposed to the center of gravity of the universe. But your center of gravity is unified by the center of gravity of the universe. Now you must understand clearly where you come from and where you go. You come from the center of gravity and you go to the center of gravity. If you think of going somewhere else, you'll have trouble." *Buddha Is the Center of Gravity,* Lama Foundation, 1974.

The Spiralic Concept of Man

by Herman Aihara

It was 1940 when World War II started and I met George Ohsawa for the first time. His lecture on "East and West" from a macrobiotic view interested me in studying more about his thought. I started to read all his writings, both magazines and books. However, I was not yet on the macrobiotic diet because my parents were against it.

I became serious about studying macrobiotics when I almost lost my mind as a result of my former wife's suicide. I went to Ohsawa's school to study the macrobiotic philosophy more deeply, because I thought instinctively that Ohsawa's teaching would help me overcome my depression.

At that time Ohsawa was forty-seven and had just been released from the Allied Forces' prison. Since he had just finished writing a small book called *The Order of the Universe,* he was giving lectures on the spiralic concept of the Order of the Universe. It was this concept that helped me to understand who I was, to recover from my depression, cross the Pacific ocean, and overcome all difficulties with joy and happiness. I think Ohsawa's concept of "man and the universe" unifies man and the universe, mind and matter. Therefore, this concept leads from dualism to monism. In this sense, this small booklet of Ohsawa's is the most important of all the books he wrote, as he himself said.

The following article is one of my applications of the concept of the Order of the Universe. This understanding is what led me to a monistic way of thinking, a course which has made my life a simple and happy one. I am sure that if you learn this book well and understand its concept, you can achieve a much happier and healthier life.

What is man? Since the early ages of civilization man has been defined metaphysically, but not physically. Scholars and thinkers gave their thoughts on man's morals, man's faith, but nothing about the physical or biological origin of man. They mostly considered the value of man, but not the origin, future, or function of man.

In *The Great Ideas, A Syntopicon of Great Books of the Western World* (Encyclopedia Britannica, Inc., 1952), editor Mortimer Adler writes: "Ancient poetry and history contain many myths of man's kinship with the gods. The heroes trace their lineage back to the gods. Through them or through the progenitors of the race, man conceives himself as of divine descent, at least, as having more affinity with the immortal gods than with all other earthbound things."

In Eastern thought, man as well as animals, plants, and things are all considered *maya* – illusionary things because they are not eternal.

"Real man is oneness and infinity, the omnipresent Spirit. And the apparent man is only an imitation of that real man. In this sense the mythologies are true, that the apparent man, however great he may be, is only a dim reflection of the real man, which is beyond. The real man, the Spirit being beyond cause and effect, not bound by time and space, must therefore be free. He was never bound, and could not be bound. The apparent man, the reflection, is limited by time, space and causation, and is therefore bound." (From *Jnana-Yoga* by Swami Vivekananda, Advaita Ashrama, 1915.)

Such a metaphysical concept of man had been the leading thought of many civilizations for thousands of years. Ancient peoples were very yang physically and because of a vegetarian diet their thought tended to be metaphysical or spiritual. They were distinguished in astronomy, cosmology and metaphysics. However, because of a change of climate and foods, man changed in his way of thinking toward one that was more analytical, empirical, and materialistic.

Modern-day people neither believe nor understand something they can't see or touch. Therefore, for them the old concept of man is inconceivable. In the past couple of hundred years distinguished observers of nature and great materialistic thinkers have appeared one after the other. Their findings and theories started to change the concept of man as well as the view of the universe. Two of the most important of these are Karl Marx and Charles Darwin, both of the 19th century. Karl Marx's theories on economics divided the world into the categories of capital and labor. He says in his *Capital* (*Great Books of the Western World*, Encyclopedia Britannica, Inc., 1952): "Man himself, viewed as the impersonation of labor power, is a natural object, a thing, although a living conscious thing, and labor is the manifestation of this power residing in him."

Charles Darwin's theory of evolution also divided the world in two, that is to say, between men who believe in the image of God and men who believe their origin is from the apes. He says in *The Origin of Species* (*Great Books of the Western World,* Encyclopedia Britannica, Inc., 1952): "I cannot pretend to throw the least light on such abstruse problems. The mystery of the beginning of all things is insoluble by us; and I for one must be content to remain an agnostic." Darwin's presentation of his theory, based on accumulated indisputable evidence and using natural selection as the mechanism of evolution, convinced and influenced people's views on the origin and concept of man. His influence was so great that churches immediately viewed the Darwinian theses as dangerous to religion and roused a storm of opposition.

One of the first clashes between the Church and science on the issue of Darwinism took place in Oxford at a meeting of the British Association for the Advancement of Science on June 30, 1860. Darwinism was the theme of the conference. Bishop Samuel Wilberforce was the prosecutor of Darwinism. At the conclusion of his forceful address, which he believed had smashed Darwin's theory, the Bishop turned to Thomas Huxley, an English biologist (1825–1896) and defender of Darwin, who was sitting on the platform with him. "I should like to ask Professor Huxley," the Bishop said cynically, "is it on your grandfather's or your grandmother's side that the ape comes in?"

Huxley is reported to have said: "A man has no reason to be ashamed of having an ape for his grandfather. If there were an ancestor whom I should feel shame in recalling, it would be a man of restless and versatile nature, who, not content with success in his own sphere of activity, plunges into scientific questions with which he has no real acquaintance, only to obscure them by an aimless rhetoric, and distract the attention of his hearers from the point at issue by eloquent digressions and skilled appeals to religious prejudice."

Such disputes and rage between religion and science continued for years. Religion neither convinces nor understands science, and vice versa. Why? There is no principle, view, or concept that encompasses both religion and science.

From the standpoint of macrobiotics, Darwin's theory of "survival of the fittest" is a hypothesis because it doesn't explain the mechanism of how species adapt to their environment. *The Origin of Species* is based on three premises and two deductions drawn from those premises.

The first premise is that all living things vary, or differ from one another. The second is that all living species tend to increase in geometric ratio. The third is that the numbers of species tend nevertheless to remain fairly constant.

From these premises Darwin draws two deductions: One is that there is a struggle for existence, and the second is that in that struggle only the fittest survive. However, Darwin didn't explain why all living things vary, or why living species tend to increase in geometric ratio. Since he couldn't explain the reason for such premises, his deductions remain hypotheses.

Macrobiotically speaking, the secret of species' fitness or adaptation lies in their foods. And food also is the cause of the variation of species. Eating different foods will cause different characters, shapes, colors, tendencies, behaviors, etc. Since every food is different, so are all living things different. Without foods there could be no life on this planet. This fact is so obvious that all scientists, including Darwin, have overlooked it.

This failure to consider foods has caused many misunderstandings in biology. For example, modern biology teaches that some African tribes are tall because tall men are cooler and better suited to the hot African climate, and therefore such tall tribes survived.

This thinking sounds right, but if we examine it carefully, it is childish thinking. First of all, there is an assumption that there were shorter tribes as well as taller ones, and that the shorter tribes died away because they didn't fit into the environment. Then we are left with the question of what made shorter tribes shorter and taller tribes taller. You may say that in the beginning there were taller and shorter tribes just by chance. Then you have to explain why no such chance exists today.

There is similar thinking on the part of modern molecular biology, which says that man is made up of organs and muscles, which in turn are made up of cells. Cells are made of cell membranes, mitochondria, etc. These, in turn, are made of protein, DNA, and RNA (a high molecular compound), which are made of amino acids, nucleotids, and these are reduced finally to atoms.

Molecular biology has found that DNA can copy the arranging DNA bases (there are a total of five bases, three of which make one amino acid). Those amino acids, in turn, make up protein. Therefore, DNA can produce protein as coded in the original DNA. However, it seems to me nobody is asking how the original coding was made in the DNA, such as arranging DNA bases in an orderly way so that they produce 20 amino acids.

According to science the appearance of original DNA is by chance, in the same way that it explains the origin of species. Therefore, however well molecular biology may explain the production of protein, cells, and man, its explanations are only hypotheses, because they do not explain the origin.

According to macrobiotics the evolution of species is the evolution of foods. (See *Macrobiotic Monthly,* Oroville, vol. 8, #12, and *The Order of the Universe,* [magazine] Boston, June, 1967.) According to Dr. Patrick M. Hurlay, the Earth was formed about 4.5 billion years ago and the stable mantle of the Earth was formed about 2.8 billion years ago. At that time the Earth was covered by water. Food, therefore, was water.

About three billion years ago bacteria, and then a little later algae, evolved from water, probably as a result of the atomic reaction of carbon, nitrogen, oxygen and hydrogen with the help of various radiations. From these developed the more complicated organisms such as sponges, around 900 million years ago. Then shellfish and primitive fish, such as plankton, arose around 425 million years ago. Some of these started to eat other fish and became more yang.

Around 360 million years ago the water receded and land appeared. Many species died, but the fishes and plants that were more yang and therefore capable of adapting to the new environment survived as land plants and amphibians.

Around 255 million years ago ferns and mosses grew on the land. Then reptiles, insects and spiders arose. The climate became warmer and warmer; then plants and animals became bigger (more yin). Dinosaurs and huge ferns inhabited the Earth at this time (200 million years ago). Then the climate started to cool and mammals evolved. As the climate became colder, carnivorous mammals and birds evolved. Some yin mammals escaped to the trees avoiding being eaten by carnivorous mammals. This is the beginning of monkeys and primates about 75 million years ago. Through eating mainly fruits and nuts (yin foods) they developed intelligence.

Some of those fruitarians found grains on the ground and started to eat them. This gave them a more upright posture and more intelligence. As a result they developed the use of hands, and *homo faber* evolved. One day some of the *homo faber* group discovered how to make and use fire. This was the beginning of *homo sapiens*.

EVOLUTION OF ANIMALS
Time Units in Millions of Years

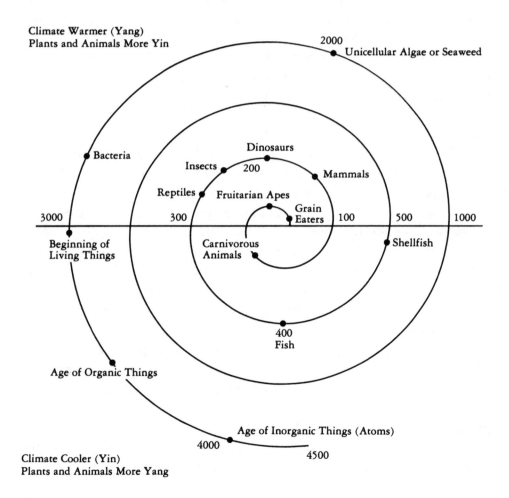

The above diagram is based on Ashley Montagu's "Time Scale of the Appearance of Various Lives" from *The Human Connection* (McGraw-Hill Book Company, 1979). Contrary to the usual diagram in the shape of a tree, I have made it in spiralic form in order to clarify the theory of evolution as understood by the Unique Principle. (The spiralic diagram of plant evolution is shown in *Macrobiotic Monthly,* vol. 8, #12; however, that diagram needs some revision.)

In this diagram the upper part indicates hotter or warmer, that is, yang climate on the Earth. Therefore, life appearing on the upper part tends to be yin (such as cold-blooded animals, or animals without blood, or reptiles).

In contrast to the upper part, the lower part of the diagram indicates a more yin climate, that is to say, a colder climate. Therefore, life appearing on the lower part of the diagram tends to be yang (stronger, warm-blooded animals). For example, unicellular algae, seaweed, dinosaurs and fruitarians appear in the upper part and they are yin. On the other hand, fishes, amphibians, and carnivorous animals appear in the lower part of the diagram and they are yang.

Thus modern science tells us that man evolved from unicellular organisms which appeared on the Earth about 3 billion years ago. The evolution of man passed through the stages of fish, amphibian, carnivorous animal, fruitarian ape, grain-eating ape, and finally to modern man.

Strangely enough, our life passes through these 3 billion years of evolution in only a year or so. The beginning of our life is unicellular – which begins with conception resulting from the union of an egg and a sperm. The next stage we pass through is that of fish and amphibian. At this time we are fed solely by our mother's blood; hence, we are carnivorous.

Then birth follows. We learn to crawl. We drink our mother's milk. This stage parallels that of the fruitarian ape. Then we start to eat grains and stand up. This is the stage of *homo faber.* The last stage arrives when man has learned how to use fire. This gives him the freedom of surviving in a colder climate and of enjoying a wider selection of foods. This, in turn, contributes to his being a grain-eater and helps to develop his intelligence.

Let us think one step further. In our daily life we eat two or three times a day, or even five times. Whatever foods we eat, they are decomposed by the various digestive juices and are transformed into blood plasma in our intestinal walls. And then later this plasma is transformed into red cells and body cells. Another way to say it is that we are transmuting from vegetable to animal in twenty-four hours every day. In other words, the three billion years' of evolution is taking place every day in our bodies. This is not an easy job to do in such a short time. This is the reason why we have so many different kinds of human beings on this Earth:

> Man like a fish and amphibian: His action is a reflection of sense stimulation. He is not using the big brain in his actions.
> Man like a reptile: He is lazy.
> Man like an insect: He is busy all the time.
> Man like a carnivore: He is cautious and aggressive.
> Man like a monkey: He is funny and cunning.
> Man like a bird: He likes to show off.

These are all on their way in the evolution of man, but they have not reached their goal yet. As members of the human species each has developed physically, but not yet psychologically or spiritually.

As I have already stated, the evolution of three billion years is taking place every day in our bodies. How can we transform three billion years of evolution in just a day or so?

In our three billion years of transformation or evolution we acquired some tools. The first one is the introduction of enzymes. Every living thing produces its own enzymes which promote decomposition, chemical reaction, and composition of its foods.

The second tool is the ability to transmute hemoglobin from chlorophyl. In short, the transmutation from magnesium (Mg) to iron (Fe). This transmutation happens like this: $Mg(24) + O_2 (16 \times 2) \rightarrow Fe(56)$. (Here the numbers inside the parentheses are the atomic weights.) In order for the atom magnesium to combine with two atoms of oxygen, the magnesium must be very yang.

Exercise, fire (cooking), salt (cooking with miso, soy sauce, or salt) and aging (such as pickling) are all yangizing factors. The lack of such factors in our eating and living situation will result in an anemic condition. A meat-eater will get plenty of hemoglobin from meat; therefore, he will not be anemic even though he eats large quantities of vegetables and fruits without fire, salt, and pickling. However, a vegetarian must yangize his vegetables or he will have a shortage of iron (Fe).

The third contribution that evolution has made is that the blood cells are very close to body cells in the ratio of potassium (K) to sodium (Na). According to my study, the ratio K/Na by weight in regular vegetables, plasma, blood cells and body cells is:

Regular vegetables	5/1 – 40/1
Blood plasma	1/10 – 1/16
Blood cells	5/1 – 10/1
Body cells	5/1 – 10/1

In this chart only the blood plasma is different from the others and it is yang; the others are comparatively yin.

Since our food consists of vegetables, the beginning of man's transmutation is the vegetal world, which is the Sixth World or Second Heaven in Ohsawa's spiralic concept of the world. This food passes through all the digestive organs. The bile from the liver increases the contents of sodium and changes digested food to plasma in the intestine wall. This yang plasma attracts yin oxygen and transmutes sodium to potassium. And the result is an increase of potassium:

$$Na(23) + O(16) \rightarrow K(39)$$

Potassium-rich plasma changes into red blood cells. Lacking DNA, red blood cells are like a virus, entering body cells and supplying them with oxygen and nutrients. Red blood cells which acquire DNA are changed into body cells.

In other words, plasma acquires oxygen and transmutes into blood cells and then into body cells, as mentioned above. Evolution itself ends with the plasma; our evolution, however, continues further.

Our evolution continues in the area of mentality or spirituality. This is our spiritual development. This spiritual development, according to Ohsawa, consists in the seven levels of judgment. The seventh level of spirituality is Infinity, our original starting point. When we reach Infinity (or all-embracing Love) then our evolution is complete.

Therefore, the origin of man and DNA both originate from Infinity or, to use the old name, God. In short, the origin of DNA which scientists have failed to find, is Infinity or God. In this regard, Ohsawa's concept of *The Order of the Universe* can lead us to a monistic view in our understanding of the *origin* of all things and in this way save us from much confusion.

TURNING POINT OF EVOLUTION
– BODY TO MIND –

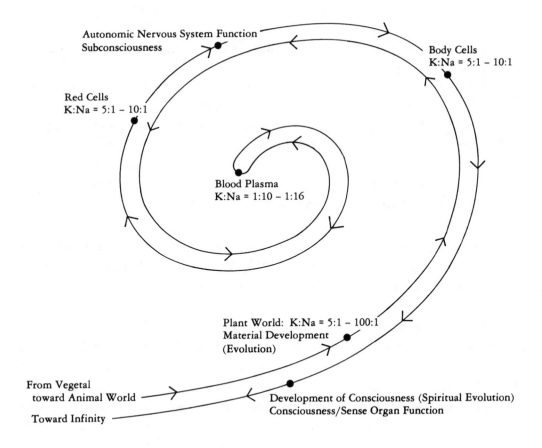

Autonomic Nervous System Function
Subconsciousness

Body Cells
K:Na = 5:1 – 10:1

Red Cells
K:Na = 5:1 – 10:1

Blood Plasma
K:Na = 1:10 – 1:16

Plant World: K:Na = 5:1 – 100:1
Material Development
(Evolution)

From Vegetal
toward Animal World

Development of Consciousness (Spiritual Evolution)
Consciousness/Sense Organ Function

Toward Infinity

Recently on a speaking tour in Sweden I lectured on the subject of psychological and spiritual sicknesses. This subject is one of the many applications of Ohsawa's spiralic explanation of the Order of the Universe. I write it here so that you also may benefit from this great concept of *The Order of the Universe*.

The Buddha taught people how to overcome sickness and suffering. He divided physiological sicknesses into four kinds: They are the sicknesses caused by living, old age, illness and death. He divided psychological sicknesses or sufferings into four also:

1. Meeting those we don't like.
2. Separation from those we love.
3. Frustration at not getting what we want.
4. Suffering arising from stress caused by ego emotions.

According to the Buddha there are 404 physical sicknesses and 84,000 psychological sicknesses. In our highly civilized world of today there must be many more sicknesses than during the Buddha's time.

I divide psychological sicknesses into two, yin and yang. Our emotions swing between yin emotions and yang emotions. This can be described as a seesaw:

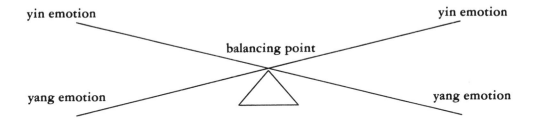

Yin Emotion	Balancing Point	Yang Emotion
Indifference	Contentedness	Jealousy
Inferiority	Confidence	Overconfidence
Worry	Peace of Mind	Anger
Whining	Responsibility	Complaining
Sadness	Happiness	Excessive joy
Doubt or Fear	Faith	Arrogance
No opinion	Firmness	Stubborn

Since the extremities of yin or yang emotions are the psychological sicknesses, the cure for these sicknesses is to move toward the balancing point. The balancing point doesn't move while the extremities swing from yin to yang and vice versa. So such a balancing point exists at the seventh level of judgment, as Ohsawa says in *The Book of Judgment* (George Ohsawa Macrobiotic Foundation, 1980) and as I have mentioned in my explanation of the Spiral of Man.

How can we attain the seventh level of judgment?

As I wrote in the preceding section, when man's evolution has reached its terminus, that is to say, when blood plasma (the most yang part of man) has been formed, man is ready to begin his spiritual development or evolution.

The first level in his development is mechanical judgment which includes instinct, sexual love, appetite, thirst, etc. This level is reached a couple of weeks after birth.

The second level is the development of the sense organs, called sensorial judgment, by which colors, sounds, smells, tastes, and body sensations can be distinguished. This level can be reached within a month following birth.

The third level is emotional judgment which starts functioning about a couple of months after birth. This level includes judgments of like or dislike, love or hate, resentment or jealousy, worry or anger, sadness or joy, etc.

Around the age of four we start showing intellectual judgment, that is to say, a love of knowledge, inquiring about the meanings, causes, or the characteristics of things, both existent and non-existent. Some even begin to distinguish numbers. For example, some children want two cakes instead of one, which means they know that two is better than one, or that two can give them more satisfaction. This is the fourth level of judgment.

The fifth level of judgment is called social or economic. This level begins around the age of six. At this age children are conformists. They want to do what others do. When my kids started elementary school my wife gave them whole wheat sandwiches with peanut butter. But they wouldn't eat them at school because the other kids would say "icky-icky." My kids wanted to do what others do. This is social judgment. If people stayed at this level, world unity would be easily achieved.

But about the age of fifteen kids begin to want to act differently from others. They don't want to be like everyone else. This also is social judgement, but expressed differently.

Around the age of twenty, one arrives at the sixth level of judgment, moral judgment, which is about choosing good or bad, right or wrong, etc. This level of judgment leads us to religions. For example, Zen Buddhism thinks that man is good and that only his mind or thinking is clouded. So if he wipes away the cloud his Buddha nature will be revealed. The Shin sect of Buddhism, on the other hand, thinks that man's nature is bad, that it is greedy, jealous, lazy, ignorant, etc. Therefore he must ask for the Buddha's help and mercy in order to reach happiness.

Such differences in man's evaluation of the meaning of life creates different religions. Since those judgments are at a very high level, the differences between religions are difficult to resolve or bring together.

All the above six levels of judgment are antagonistic to one another and will therefore create disagreements, arguments, conflicts, emotional stress, or suffering. In order to overcome these conflicts or sufferings we must reach the seventh level of judgment, and that is the balancing point of the emotions.

Three ways to reach the seventh level of judgment are:

> 1. Visualization: The world we live in is the relative world. Our time here lasts about seventy or eighty years. Even lucky persons rarely live more than a hundred years. In this ephemeral world we think we want to be rich, famous, and happy. However, since we live in the relative world, what we have or get always turns into its opposite. In other words, rich changes to poor, famous to infamous, happy to unhappy, healthy to sick, etc. Therefore, the more we hang on to the relative world the more emotional troubles we will have.
>
> If we compare the relative world with the infinite world we find that, viewed from Infinity, nothing changes; nothing in the absolute world is relative.
>
> When you visualize the relative world from the infinite world you think that what you have in the relative

world is not so important or so real. As you think of the relative world as being smaller in time and space your emotions become smaller, since emotions belong only to the relative world. And when your emotions become smaller you are approaching the balancing point of the seesaw; in other words, you are nearing Infinity.

2. Diet: The macrobiotic diet is a low-fat, low-sugar, high complex carbohydrate diet, emphasizing whole grains, fresh vegetables, sea vegetables, a balanced sea salt, and a good balance of yin and yang, and acid and alkaline.

3. Giving up: Giving up what you have is releasing the pull of gravity that binds you to this relative world. Therefore, giving up means that your level of judgment is closer to the seventh level. Giving up is the same as reaching this level, since to give up is to reduce our ego desires (lower judgment) and enter the higher or seventh level of judgment. Therefore, giving up makes us *really* happy, not just relatively happy; it gives us real happiness, health and wealth.

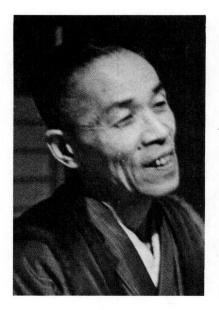

George Ohsawa (Yukikazu Sakurazawa, 1893–1966). At the age of sixteen, suffering with tuberculosis, stomach ulcers, and a host of other illnesses, he was pronounced "incurable."

Determined to get well, he began his life-long study of the ancient Indian, Chinese, and Japanese writings on the principles of natural living. He gradually came to an understanding of the physical and spiritual dynamics of health and happiness, which he termed "macrobiotics."

Ohsawa spent his life writing and lecturing in an effort to share with others this basic wisdom, long forgotten in most cultures. He is the author of over three hundred books, many of which have been translated into many languages.

Books by George Ohsawa in English

The Book of Judgment

Gandhi, the Eternal Youth

Jack and Mitie

Macrobiotic Guidebook for Living

Macrobiotics: An Invitation to Health and Happiness
 (with Herman Aihara)

Macrobiotics: The Way of Healing

The Order of the Universe

The Unique Principle

You Are All Sanpaku

Zen Macrobiotics

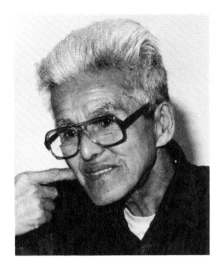

Herman Aihara was born in Arita, Japan on September 28, 1920. He first heard of Mr. Ohsawa before entering Waseda University, but it wasn't until after he graduated with a bachelor's degree in Metallurgical Engineering that he attended Ohsawa's classes and eventually decided to emigrate to the United States to teach macrobiotics.

Mr. Aihara founded, and is President of, both the George Ohsawa Macrobiotic Foundation and the Vega Study Center. With the help of his wife, Cornellia, he continues to write, publish, translate, lecture, and spread macrobiotic thinking throughout the world.

Books by Herman Aihara

Acid and Alkaline

Basic Macrobiotics

Kaleidoscope

Learning from Salmon

Macrobiotics: An Invitation to Health and Happiness
    (with George Ohsawa)

The works of George Ohsawa and Herman and Cornellia Aihara, as well as a complete book list of macrobiotic titles, are available from:

George Ohsawa Macrobiotic Foundation
1511 Robinson Street
Oroville, California 95965
(916) 533-7702